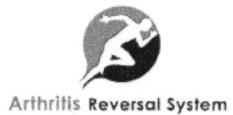

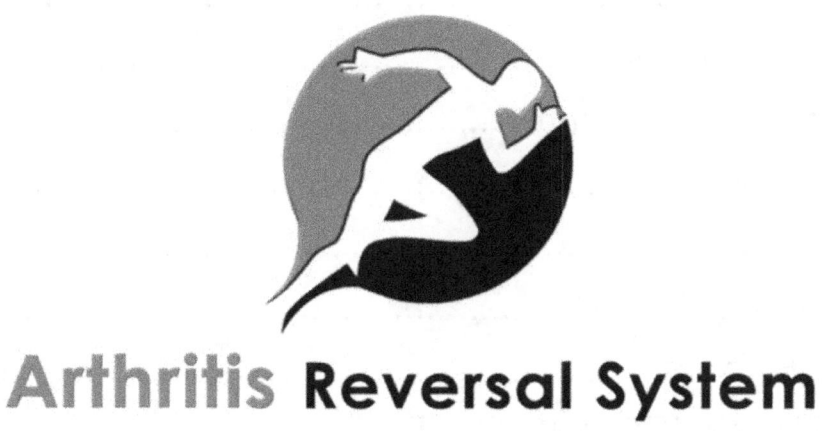

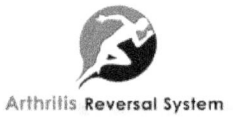

Table of Contents

INTRODUCTION 6
    Anatomy 8
    Inflammation 10
    NSAIDs 11
    Cholesterol Drugs 14
    High Blood Pressure 18
    Meniscus & Blood Supply 23
    What can you Take? 26
    Heal the Gut 30
    Fast Pain Relief NOW 32
    Looking Forward 36
ARTHRITIS REVERSING DIET 40
    Water 43
    Meat 45
    Heartburn Prevention 48
    pH 53
BREAKFAST 53
    Dairy 55
LUNCH 58
DINNER 61
SUMMARY 64
REGENERATIVE EXERCISES 70
EXERCISE 71
    Muscle Imbalances 76

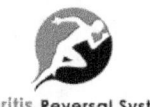

Anatomy	80
Golgi Tendon Organ	83
NSAIDs	84
Start Where You Are	87
Safe Lifting	91
Range of Motion	95
Can I Tell You a Secret?	98
SELF-TALK	**102**
Vision Board	105
100 Ways to a Better Life	108
NLP	112
Breathe	114
SUMMARY	**118**
THE NERVOUS SYSTEM	**124**
What's the Connection?	128
New Way of Thinking	132
Alternative Source of Brain Power	135
Chronic Stress	137
7 Questions	139
Additional Studies	141
MDs Don't Look for what they Can't Fix	144
SUMMARY & CALL TO ACTION	**145**

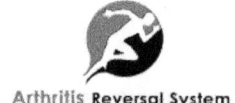

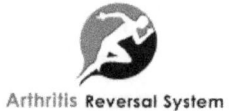

THE TRUTH

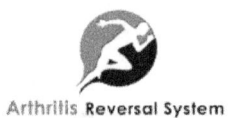

INTRODUCTION

Arthritis and drugs. Now, this is going to be kind of like Basic Common Sense. I know it's going to sound crazy because arthritis... it's the plague! It happens when you're old. No, it's not true. Joints are brilliant and what's neat is, you know how mom said, "Don't crack your knuckles. They're going to swell up and cause damage?" No, the British medical journal did a study and found out that habitual knuckle crackers, and you've got to love the Brits, they have a remarkable lack of arthritis.

Joints have to move to be healthy. Every time you move a joint, it pushes blood and fluid to hydrate it. This is why medications are so vital to understand. The medications get into the blood stream. They affect metabolic processes. If you realize that your body is a sea of metabolic processes including joints, all of the structures in the body are alive. I know this sounds crazy but I talk to multiple, multiple health care professionals. They come to see me. I've got orthopedic surgeons, liver specialists, pharmacists; I've got hundreds of nurses. Nurses get the big picture. God bless you, gals.

When you look at it, all the tissue in the body is alive. For all of the tissue in the body to be alive, you have to do a couple of things with the cells. They've got to take in nutrients, they've got to produce proteins and they've got to eliminate waste products. That's every cell. That means the meniscus has to do that. That means the cartilage has to do it. That means the bones have to do it.

Notes

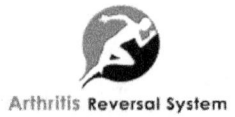

Anatomy

Now I'm going to give you a quick anatomy lesson. What joints are, and this is pretty much most of the joints in the body, they're two bones joined together surrounded by a joint capsule. And that joint capsule has a filtration system and it gives a super filtrate a blood called synovial fluid. The synovial fluid gives nutrients to the cartilage. Every time you open and close that joint you create a negative pressure. Bam! Synovial fluid comes rushing in. You create a positive pressure. Bam! It's squeezed out. You get this pumping action in there to allow the cells to get healthy nutrients.

Now, you're thinking, "Hey, wait a second! If joints have to move and joints have to have healthy blood supply, what causes arthritis?" I'm glad you asked because what causes arthritis is:

- ✓ toxic blood
- ✓ poor motion
- ✓ poor nerve supply

All the joints have nerve supply. In fact, the nerves that supply the joints, supply the muscles, supply the skin and supply everything. You have to have a healthy nervous system.

Now, when we look at this, we've got the two bones coming together surrounded by a joint capsule. If there's damage to the joint, the body is going to inflame. I know. Inflammation is part of the body's repair process.

Notes

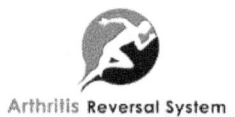

Inflammation

It's vital that you understand there are two types of inflammation. One type is systemic inflammation. That's when your whole body inflames, that's bad. That's the source of most diseases; it's the source of adrenal fatigue, it's the source of thyroid disorders and it's the source of most cancers.

Systemic inflammation? Bad. We're going to talk about systemic inflammation because you've got to understand the difference in order to realize how to reverse arthritis and how to get healthy joints.

Local inflammation is good. This is what causes the tissues to be repaired. I've got a lot of experience on this. Okay? I was run over by a car, had both of my legs broken, my sternum fractured, my skull fractured, my front teeth knocked out, liver bruised, heart bruised- wait, no. My heart was bruised back in the fourth grade. No, it was bruised at this accident too.

What you've got to look at is that I've got experience because discs do re-grow; they do regenerate. The way you do it is to clean the blood, healthy nerve supply and have healthy motion, so this is vital. What the medical profession today doesn't understand, and not just the medical profession, we're talking the health experts in the gym, okay, your corner grocer, the cleaners you go to. It's pervasive because the population is educated that inflammation is bad.

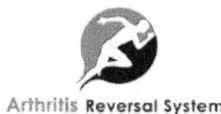

NSAIDs

I saw a commercial the other day,

"Take Advil for peak performance on the golf course."

I'm going, "Oh, no!" Advil is in a class of drugs called nonsteroidal anti-inflammatories (NSAIDs). Now, that's Advil, ibuprofen and Motrin. Tylenol is not a nonsteroidal anti-inflammatory but it has a similar effect. When you look at the research behind it, this is crazy. Nonsteroidal anti-inflammatories, the way they work in the body is they inhibit proteoglycan production. That's the building block of cartilage.

Think about this. You have got all of the joints in the body. Two bones coming together surrounded by a joint capsule. It starts to inflame because the body has damage to the joint, so the body is trying to inflame it in order to regenerate it. Then somebody is going to give you a drug to make you comfortable to stop the repair process? Think about this. If local inflammation is a body's repair process, why is the public and the medical profession brainwashed to think that it's bad?

Well, you've got to think there are only two countries that allow DTC, direct-to-consumer advertising, for pharmaceutical products: New Zealand and America. What are the two countries with the highest cancer rates? New Zealand and America. Okay, so it's a little bit crazy.

When we look at this, nonsteroidal anti-inflammatories inhibit the building block of cartilage so that means they're actually destroying the joints so they make you comfortable while your joints are being destroyed. Because we've got the nonsteroidal anti-

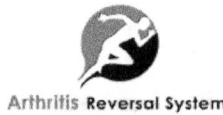

inflammatories, let's look at the other drugs that are out there that are causing destruction of the joints. I know when you look at this, arthritis pain medications, I want you comfortable. There are a lot of things out there that you can take to increase that healing process, which is inflammation.

I know I can see it right now, a bunch of skulls are about to break open because this information is so rare. Yes, I'm going to give you some advice on how to increase the inflammatory response to the joints so that you can regenerate cartilage and regenerate meniscus and heal. Heck, you even build new synovial fluid. You build new synovial membranes. Your body is a sea of metabolic processes.

Notes

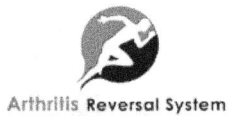

Cholesterol Drugs

That leads us to the next class of drugs that's absolutely deadly: cholesterol drugs. I encourage everybody to watch the ***Statin Nation***. Cholesterol is the building product of virtually everything your body makes. Nearly every cell in your body has a cell wall composed of cholesterol. Your brain is composed of cholesterol. Your adrenals are the pharmacy of the body. They produce every glucocorticosteroid, every mineral-corticosteroid and sex hormone. They protect you from cancer. They're vital.

Your adrenals produce the greatest anti-inflammatory known to mankind. It's called cortisol. I know, I know. You've heard of cortisol that it's a stress hormone, and it is. It's also vital to the immune system. See what cortisol is, is it's an anti-inflammatory that's going to slow down the inflammatory process. *But it can only be used a short time.* What does the body use to build cortisol? It uses cholesterol.

If you go and you've been diagnosed with high cholesterol, I've got to tell you that's not a disease. **75%** of all people who have a heart attack have lower to normal cholesterol. You've been fed a lie that cholesterol is bad and it's actually used for tissue repair. The only reason that cholesterol could be a sign of bad is if you have a lot of tissue damage, systemic inflammation which again, we know that causes disease and cancers and joint destruction.

But if you have high cholesterol for long periods of time it means that you have high stress or tissue damage. To lower the cholesterol, that's like putting a black piece of tape over the light on the dashboard. That's just foolish. I encourage everyone to watch the movie ***Statin Nation***. It's out of England and it details

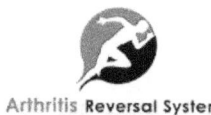

out exactly the scam of getting cholesterol medications into the population. By the way, Lipitor was the first drug to cross the **$15 billion a year mark**. That's right. Super profitable and super evil.

Nonsteroidal anti-inflammatories, Advil, Aleve, Motrin, ibuprofen, all of those. Do you know how Tylenol works? Nope. Neither do they. This is the weird part. When you look at all medications, Tylenol is really fun and you need to decipher the language. You've got to remember the system is not laid out for easy access to information.

One of the best sites I've seen is *rxlist.com*. You go on there, you type in the name of drugs and it will tell you everything about the drug. And I mean way more information than you could possibly need when you look up clinical pharmacology. But I encourage you to go on there because, see, the medical profession is providing just what their education allowed them.

The pharmaceutical industry has been donating and funding medical education since the '20s. The doctors today, they take very little anatomy, very little physiology, and that's at the beginning of the education process. Then they're taught symptom-therapy, symptom-therapy, and symptom-therapy. When you go in there, the doctors are trained to memorize and regurgitate information. If you say a certain condition, arthritis. Bam! Anti-inflammatories. Arthritis medications. Naproxen.

All of these different drugs our there that they have, but how do they actually work? When you look up the clinical pharmacology behind Tylenol, Tylenol is not only the number one prescribed drug in America, it's also the deadliest drug in America. You look at the clinical pharmacology it says the mechanism action remains elusive or unknown. Yes, flowery terms but it doesn't make sense.

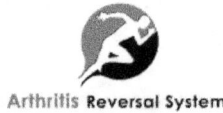

If you have common sense, this isn't going to sound appropriate to you to provide a chemical that destroys joint cartilage and is the deadliest drug in America for temporary relief of pain? But remember, this information on this video is to allow you to heal the joints, to regenerate and renew and restore to get those joints that are damaged with pain to have them regenerate. Now, a chemical slows down that process.

Notes

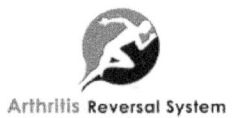

High Blood Pressure

Now, let's look at another crazy thing. High blood pressure. Okay, now, when we do our videos, and we just did a video on cancer, we found that if you take a calcium channel blocker for ten years, your risk of cancer has tripled or quadrupled depending on the type of cancer it is. If you take a beta blocker, which is another type of blood pressure drug, your risk of heart attacks increases.

But let's look at this. Remember, joints are two bones coming together surrounded by a joint capsule. That joint capsule has blood that's filtered through it, so the health of the blood is vital. Let's say that you have arteries that used to be as big and healthy. Let's say they're a little bit small or damaged. Let's say that we eat hamburgers or fast food at every meal. That damages the lining of the arteries. Let's say that you don't understand that genetically modified foods, I know, excuse me if you're watching this from Europe this isn't going to make sense.

A lot of the genetically modified foods in Europe are outlawed, okay? Because they know they're bad. If you're watching this in Europe as well as China and Russia and most every country on the planet, the public can actually go into the store and read the package and it will say "Non-GMO" or "GMO", in this country it's not even legal to *label* the food if it's GMO. Genetically Modified Organisms actually damage the lining of the arteries so that closes it down.

Now, think about this. If you have smaller arteries and you need to get the same amount of blood through it, the same amount of nutrients, what do you think has to happen to pressure in order to get the same nutrients and fluids to the joints, the organ systems, and everything? Yes, it's got to go up.

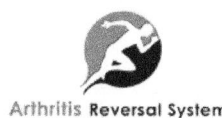

High blood pressure is not a disease. It's a clue to a damaged, stressed system. Now here's the good news: those arteries can open up. They can be cleaned because, remember, they're living tissue. I encourage you to either read my book, "*How to Correct High Blood Pressure Without Medications*" or just use some common sense. There's a great video called "*Eating.*" It talks about a plant based diet can actually clean the arteries.

There are machines out there that cause you to deep breathe. It's called meditation. Just deep breathing 15 minutes a day will also help lower the blood pressure because it's oxygenating the system. But don't take blood pressure medications until you find the reason. Heck, I've had patients who were literally shot in the kidneys. They were still able to regulate their own bodily functions.

Again, most people are programmed by the television to think that their body can't regulate itself. I'm going to tell the truth right now. Your body is self-regulating and self-healing. Yes, that's right. You regulate your own cholesterol levels. You regulate your own blood pressure levels. You regulate your own cortisol or thyroid and stomach acids. I've got to tell you, if I smell broccoli, do you realize that that hits the area of the old brain called the olfactory bulb, which hits the limbic system, which hits the Vagus nerve, that sends the signal down and my stomach produces an acid just designed to break down that broccoli. It's true.

I want you to start appreciating that your body has physiologic processes that if you change that physiology with a chemical, the outcome is really poor. What are the side effects of blood pressure medications? We're talking brain damage, dementia, arthritis, increased inflammation, joint pain and headaches. Because what happens?

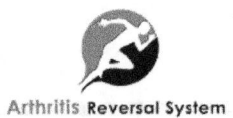

This is going to be a weird concept because I'll get educated people in and I'll say, "You're taking a drug to lower pressure. Does that help the pump or does that slow it down?" Do you know that most people say, "I don't know; I'm not a doctor,"? I know. I want to smack them, "No." You can't hit patients; that's bad. But how do you get the common sense in there?

Okay, you're taking a drug that slows down or lowers the pressure. Does that help oxygen and nutrients? And does it help eliminate waste products? No. And this is why. Remember, this video is for arthritis. I'm talking about blood pressure, cholesterol, nonsteroidal anti-inflammatories. That's right. You have to clean the blood. You have to have healthy blood in order to regenerate the joints.

Find out why the doctor is prescribing it and, honestly, if the doctor is prescribing nonsteroidal inflammatories, if they're providing cholesterol medications or if they're actually telling you to take a blood pressure drug, you've got to find another doctor. You're going to find a doctor that realizes the basics, the stuff that every other doctor learned in school: the body is self-regulating and self-healing. I know. Okay. That's a basic concept.

Now, blood pressure drugs, cholesterol drugs, anti-inflammatory drugs: all of those *decrease the body's ability to heal the joints*. Now, we have to look at something that's a little bit more important because I don't want you to have joint pain. I want you to regenerate the joints healthy and strong. We understand that the medications are bad. We understand that the health of the blood is vital. We understand that the joints are two bones coming together surrounded by a joint capsule. That joint capsule is filled with synovial fluid that nutrifies and gives health and it allows the cells inside of the joint to do this thing cells need to do. They need to produce proteins, eliminate waste products and actually live. Take in nutrients.

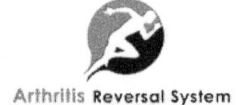

Notes

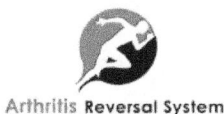

Meniscus & Blood Supply

A lot of people will say, "But meniscus doesn't have a blood supply. It can't regenerate." Okay, I understand this. I understand this is what a lot of doctors are telling you. When we look at just the knee joint itself, and we're going to cover this in future videos on how to regenerate meniscus.

You got this biggest joint in the body. You've got a tibia on the bottom. You've got this giant femur on the top and it spins and turns. So right now, what am I standing on? I'm standing on my tibia. Okay, now I'm doing this to demonstrate there's a tremendous amount of pressure that I'm putting on. Do you think blood vessels would survive that type of trauma? No. What your design is, you've got meniscus on the outside that has a blood supply, you've got meniscus on the inside that doesn't have a blood supply.

I was trying to explain this to a doctor. I said, "Yes, it doesn't have a blood supply. Why? Because the blood vessels would be crushed. Where does it get its nutrients?"

And he started to think and think and he said, "Get its nutrients? No, it doesn't have a blood supply."

And I said, "Well, is it living cells or dead cells?"

"Well, they're alive."

"Well, if they're alive are they 53, 54 years old on my body?"

"Well, I never thought of it that way."

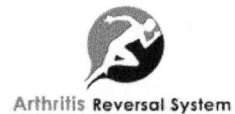

Start! Start thinking about that because remember meniscus can regenerate, ligaments can regenerate, and they get their blood supply or they get their nutrients through blood supply that's filtered through the synovial membrane. Okay, now we've got to talk about this because we're going to cover the exercises in video 3 and we're going to cover the nervous system in video 5. Now, let's talk about what you can take.

Notes

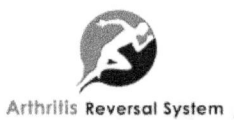

What can you Take?

First off, you've got to look at all of the medications you're taking, talk to a medical health care professional, get your body healthy so you don't require the drugs. That's right. Healthy people don't require medications. And diseases can be reversed. And I'm talking Irritable Bowel Syndrome, Crohn's Disease, all of these digestive system disorders have to be repaired. How many people are taking medications that will cause leaky gut?

And again, we've got to talk about the health of the blood. The health of the blood goes back down to digestion. When you're looking at digestion, when you're smelling that broccoli or you're smelling that beautiful rice, and your stomach is going to produce the acid, you have to chew it, you have to swallow it, and the whole process of digestion is how your body takes those proteins, breaks them into amino acids, takes the fats, breaks them into fatty acids. It takes the carbohydrates, breaks them down into usable sugars. This process of digestion is how the nutrients get in the blood.

How they get in the joint is they go through the synovial membrane, they allow the cartilage and the structures of the joints to regenerate. *What damages digestion will damage your joints.* Yes, I said that. What damages digestion, damages joints. When you look at this, what kind of things damage digestion? Well, obviously, since digestion is a tube things that will cause leaky gut, neurotoxins, genetically modified foods, antibiotics, all of these will damage the gut. That's the bad news.

The good news is the gut heals fast. You're talking **within 30 days**. However, if you have had vaccinations, antibiotics, genetically

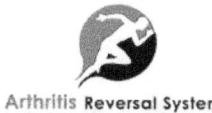

modified foods, neurotoxins in the food, such as synthetic sweeteners, aspartame, Splenda, or MSG, and you'll see there are 40 different names for MSG. The food and drug administration has dropped the ball. They're not protecting the public. That was their original intent. Now they're shields for the pharmaceutical and food industry.

You've got to look at this. If you're taking any of those, you have damage to the gut. What damage to the gut does is it allows undigested- I was going to say nutrients but really allows undigested proteins to get into the blood stream. If they get in the blood stream, the body develops a repair process. This is where antibodies come into it. Remember the two types of inflammation? Local inflammation, which is absolutely essential to healing, and it's systemic inflammation, which will kill you.

Okay, so these proteins get in the blood stream that causes systemic inflammation and if they're glutens or caseins and this is the toxic grains that we're being exposed to and the toxic dairy that we're being exposed to. There are healthy animal products out there but you don't want to have it as a mainstay of your diet. When you look at the systemic inflammatory response, that's going to close down the arteries; it's also going to negatively affect the thyroid. This is one of the organs that regulate your metabolism.

It's also going to negatively affect the adrenal glands. I mean, this is huge. So to heal the joints, you've got to heal the gut. Does that make sense? Yes, I know. This is common sense. This is what my mom told me. Well, she wasn't an anatomist but she did give me common sense. Okay. One and one is two. Okay, so you heal the gut. It takes about *30 days*. If your gut is really damaged, you're going to have to do juicing and blending. You're going to have to absolutely give up animal products, because that has toxins in it. The muscle meats have tryptophan, which slows down the thyroid.

Remember, you've got two aspects that regulate metabolic processes. If you have damaged joints, the metabolic process that I'm talking about is to cause inflammation and regenerate and renew that joint. You have to look at the thyroid and adrenals. Those are two aspects that regulate the metabolic processes that are vital to you regaining your health and reverse arthritis.

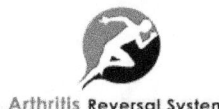

Notes

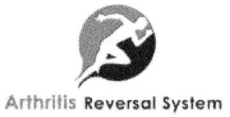

Heal the Gut

Heal the gut. Juicing and blending for about *30 days*. We have all the handouts on the juicing formulas. The type of juicer, what's the difference between juicing and blending, but what the juicing and blending basically does is it predigests the nutrients. Because remember, your gut's damaged. If you've been eating packaged foods or you've been eating genetically modified foods, or let's say you did crazy stuff like get a flu shot, okay? Or maybe you were too young to say no and they vaccinated you when you were a kid, you've got gut damage. Heal the gut about *30 to 45 days tops*, and then now look at the nutrients that we have to clean the arteries. That's right. Remember the bones coming together surrounded by synovial membrane? We need healthy blood to get to that joint in order to heal the joint and give it the nutrients.

This is where soluble fibers come in. Now, in plants there are two types of fibers: soluble and insoluble. Soluble fibers? Those are the fibers that your body can't digest that actually goes through the intestinal tract and out. Okay? That's vital. Insoluble fibers are brilliant. They're like roto-rooter to the arteries.

Think of how brilliant this is. If you take it in, you break it down; it actually starts to clean the arterial system. If you had systemic inflammation, the juicing and the blending breaks down the fibers and it cleans it. It's the most vital aspect to clean the arteries to get healthy blood to the joints.

Notes

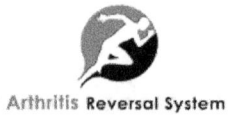

Fast Pain Relief NOW

Now, let's talk about things that we can do that we can change in our diet that are going to be vital to heal our joints. I mean, and you might say, "Yeah but my joints hurt. What do I do?" Okay, great. The first thing I want you to do if you've got joint pain, anywhere in your body, get moist heat on it. Moist heat. Okay? And why moist? Dry heat will feel good. Moist heat actually penetrates. Okay? Dr. Johnson, who was my instructor, he would always say the wetter the better, the deeper the penetration. Okay? I've got to tell you, mnemonics like that, it locks in your brain and you're going to remember that forever. I know, you're probably going to be saying that to yourself tonight.

Damp cloth in a microwave. If you don't have a microwave, heat a pot of water on the stove, heat a cloth, don't burn yourself. Be really, really careful. If you have diabetes, you're going to have loss of sensation so that can be dangerous. We have to solve the diabetes first. Wait, did I just say solve the diabetes first? Yes, that's right. You'll see in future videos.

Type 2 Diabetes, which is 95% of all *diabetes, is actually solvable in about 30 to 45 days*. I know. When you look at this, the soluble fibers you're going to clean the arteries, but moist heat on the joint, any joint that bothers you, except for the spine, don't put heat on the spine. That's a different structure. But what happens when you put heat on a joint?

And I know, I know, there are a lot of doctors out there that say, "For inflammation take an anti-flammatory and put ice on it." Let's look at that. What does ice do? Ice will decrease inflammation. Wait, didn't Dr. Bergman just say that inflammation is how the

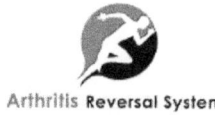

body repairs itself? Yes. You're slowing down the metabolic processes.

What would ice do? Ice slows the blood flow. Wait a second! You've got two bones coming together surrounded by a synovial membrane. Isn't blood flow important to the joint? Yes. If you've got inflammation to the joint, isn't there damage to the joint? Yes. Now, ice doesn't make sense in chronic injuries. Acute injuries, sure. Use it for 24 hours. I'm cool with that.

But for real healing you put heat on it, so what does heat do? You put heat on there and take it away. What color is your arm? It's red. That's because when you put heat on here, listen to this, your body senses that temperature differential so it increases the blood pressure and blood supply to that joint in order to equalize the temperature. Body is self-regulating, baby. You've got to love it. Let's use it. That's going to increase the blood supply.

It's also going to increase macrophage activity. This is why doctors sound really smart, because we use Latin terms. "Macro" means big; "phage" means to eat. So if I said you put moist on and that creates these cells, they're called big eaters into activity, that doesn't sound good. So let's use the Latin term, macrophage. See, the macrofages actually go in there and they chew up abnormally placed tissue. This is why when you get a bruise, bam it goes away! It's not there! Why? because that's abnormally placed blood proteins because you broke blood vessels. Well, you're going to use those babies to solve blood problems. By putting heat on there you're rushing blood that fills up, increases synovial fluid production, it also increases macrofage activity.

Because if you've got damaged joints and you're rebuilding them, you're going to have to get rid of the old bi-products. Okay? You're going to have to get rid of the old bone tissue. Yes, I said bones spurs can go away. You're going to have to get rid of the damaged parts: the damaged meniscus, the damaged ligaments, the damaged parts of the synovial membrane, even that can be repaired and that's what moist heat does.

Notes

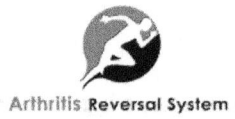

Looking Forward

In future videos, I'm going to show you how to strengthen the arm, strengthen the legs, strengthen the spine and how to move those joints because, remember, you've got to have movement. You've got to have blood supply. You've got to have nerve supply.

Now, here are some diet changes that I want you to do. Spicy foods. If you can't tolerate spicy foods, do Capsaicin or cayenne supplements. Be careful of those because they can upset your stomach. You've got to take them immediately with food. But what do spicy foods have in them? Okay, one thing is it opens up blood vessels and that causes pain relief. Because now I can start to see light bulbs go on. If you say, "Wow, increasing blood supply decreases pain. Wow, you clean the arteries that decreases pain." Why? Because you're helping the body with the inflammatory process to regenerate the joints.

And start looking at the natural things that are out there. Spices. Turmeric. Okay? One of the greatest, it's like an adapta-genetic herb where it can actually help. Many studies on it show it's better for solving cancer and tumor growth but it's also great for healing joints. And healthy spices, healthy salts, healthy vegetables, a plant based diet, all of those structures and we're going to have handouts at the end of this video you can click on that detail out nonsteroidal inflammatory foods and pain relieving foods and herbs. And that just makes sense.

The doctor of the future will not give a medication to interrupt natural metabolic processes. The doctor of the future is going to be educated and respect the body. That's what I want you to do. If you respect that the body actually has natural healing ability that it

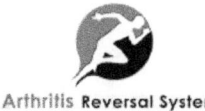

gives symptoms for a reason, you're never going to be taking a drug to interrupt those metabolic processes. You're going to correct the causes of high cholesterol, you're going to correct the situation that created high blood pressure and you're going to correct and restore and renew the joints. Healthy food, healthy blood supply, healthy arteries, healthy movement, healthy joints and if you have a doctor that's prescribing a drug for arthritis, you've got to fire him.

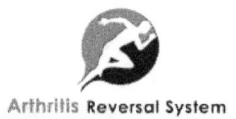

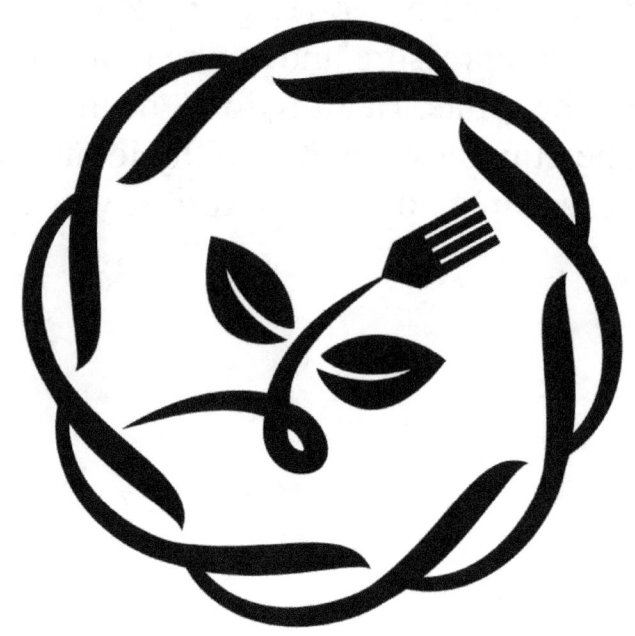

ARTHRITIS REVERSING DIET

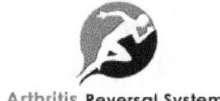

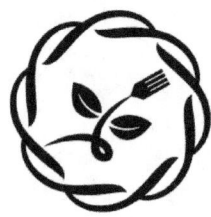

ARTHRITIS REVERSING DIET

Our next step in arthritis reversal is diet change. There's a couple of things you've got to know and I know changing your diet can be pretty intimidating because a lot of people, we have this meat addiction or fast food addiction or chocolate addiction. What I want to do, I'm going to give you a set pattern that you can change just one meal a week. One meal a week. If you do that, we're going to add to it over time.

Now there's a couple of different terms I want you to know. One of them is pH. Now, the pH of your blood. Remember blood is vital for healthy joints. Those joints, I know I'm going to repeat this again. There are two bones coming together surrounded by a joint capsule and that joint capsule has a super filtrate of blood called synovial fluid. Healthy joints, we first have to start with healthy blood.

Where does healthy blood come from? Your blood is brand new every 120 days. This means the nutrients you put in your system are absolutely essential to regenerating healthy joints. When we talk about pH and a lot of people are going to say oh, the pH is nothing. You die if your blood gets over 7.3 to 7.4 or 5. That's the range. That's true. Your body does a terrific job because if the pH of your blood goes up or down a point, you're dead.

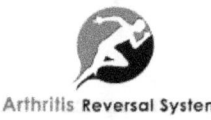

To keep alive, we actually maintain a very, very healthy pH throughout our entire life. Now, if we take in more acid forming foods or we acidify our bodies with certain practices, the body has to work harder to maintain the pH. Let me go over that again. The more acid forming foods that we put in our system such as processed foods, refined foods, smoking, alcohol, the enriched foods which are absolutely toxic. The more we acidify our body with fat, the body goes into this repair or stress mode and if it's in the repair or stress mode, it can't regenerate healthy joints, so we have to start looking at what we put in our system.

This is the first change I want you to do and you're going to have to keep a journal on this and in this journal, I want you to start marking down exactly what you're doing, what you're changing. Now, this is the biggest one and this is the hardest one. This is the number one challenge that my patients have. I tell them you have to drink water.

NOTES

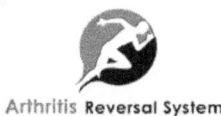

Water

The water that you put in your system is vital. You need 50 percent of your body weight in ounces a day. What that means is a 240 pound man needs 120 ounces of water minimum, but the water has to be healthy. It can't be out of a plastic container. It can't have fluoride in it. It can't have chlorine in it. That's why the number one water filter that we recommend is Doulton and you can get it at Doulton USA. It's fantastic, because it eliminates the fluoride and chlorine. (DoultonUSA.com)

If you're lucky enough to have access to spring water, that's going to be essential. Water does a couple of things. Water is a great pain reliever. Water is a great lubricant. 70 percent of your body is water so 70 percent of your meals need to be water as well. This is where plant or plant based diet is so essential.

NOTES

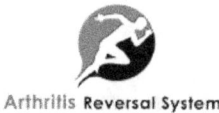

Meat

If you're addicted to meat, great. Make sure it's a healthy animal, make sure you're eating it once a week. Once a month is better. A couple of times a year is even better than that.

When you eat meat or animal products, on the muscle meat itself there's tryptophan and there's also endotoxins. The endotoxins actually cause your body to inflame, so your body has to start fighting it and the tryptophan slows down the thyroid function and when we're talking healthy diet, healthy nutrition, we have to look at the metabolic processes that actually regenerate the joints and give you the healthy building materials.

We have to start taking in, remember the body is 70 percent fluid, food has to be 70 percent fluid. Most people are dehydrated. The healthy water is ideal. If you're lucky enough to have a spring close by, spring water is the best.

There's a website called findaspring.com and I truly recommend you go there. It's almost an adventure. You'll find springs all around that are close and this is pristine water that's filtered by the earth. I totally recommend that.

Now, start the day off by drinking a *liter of water*. I know this is going to sound like a lot and if you're not used to drinking water, I got to tell you, the second half of that liter is going to start tasting like medicine, but it is. Water's going to help your brain to function quickly; it's going to help your joints to get that super filtrated blood called synovial fluid.

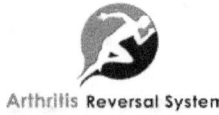

It's also going to lubricate and separate the red blood cells. The reason you want to drink it when you first get up is because at night, your body, the stomach acids are trying to digest the dinner from the night before, there's not a lot of movement of the joints during the night. Hopefully you're sleeping. When you start looking at this, if you're not moving your joints, if you're not moving the lymph fluid, in the morning you can be acidic.

What I mean by that is how many times have you gotten up and you feel like you're creaking? The tin man in the Wizard of Oz saying, "oil can!" No. You can't oil the joints with an oil can. What you can do is lubricate from the inside with water. Number one change: get water. That's going to start balancing your diet.

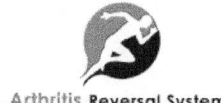

NOTES

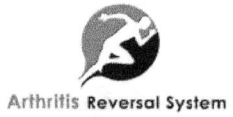

Heartburn Prevention

Now, this is also vital because you can't drink water 20 minutes before a meal, during a meal or 20 minutes after. Go on, say why. I'm going to tell you why, because you figure when you're looking at this and this is vital because it's not just diet. Whatever you put in your mouth, you have to break down and you have to break the proteins to amino acids, fats to fatty acids and carbohydrates to usable sugars.

In order to do that, you have to smell things first. When you take that rich piece of broccoli that's just been steamed and you smell it, your stomach instantly begins to produce an acid to break the proteins and fats and carbohydrates out of that broccoli so it can regenerate your tissue. Your system's fantastic.

However, if you drink water, that dilutes the acid and causes a poor digestion. We call it indigestion. I know you've heard that term. You have to start healing the gut and you have to start breaking down the proteins, fats and carbohydrates to nutrients that you can actually use.

Now if you've had a lot of gastrointestinal problems, like let's say you've been taking the little purple pill for 24 hours of relief or you're taking Tums on a regular basis. You have to heal the gut first.

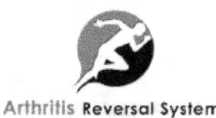

Okay, so the changes:

- Water in the morning. Absolutely a liter would be great to start the day with. A liter of healthy spring water.

- Second, no water 20 minutes before a meal, during a meal or 20 minutes after. If you have to wet your pallet, just wet it a little bit, but try not to dilute the acid.

If you've had long-term stomach issues, you have to heal the gut first. This is where blending and juicing comes in. We do an entire video series on blending, fermenting and juicing and all of those three different processes; blending, fermenting and juicing actually pre-digests the food for you because if you've had long-term medication use, long-term indigestion, long-term stress, then that means you're not going to be breaking the foods down correctly.

Scan the QR code below or enter the URL below to get videos on blending, juicing and fermenting.

http://0s4.com/r/W6Z7Al

Now, you can take or you can heal the gut in about 30 days. I don't care if you've been on antacids for 20 years. You can heal the gut in about 30 days. Why? Because that's about how long the intestinal tract takes to regenerate and heal.

If you've had major damage, start juicing and blending. I'm bringing this up because we want to work in to what's a healthy breakfast, what's a healthy lunch and what's a healthy dinner because a lot of people are losing the art of cooking.

If you're living alone, you might not want to cook for yourself. If you have a big family, you might be too tired at the end of the day to cook. I'm going to show you how to make healthy meals in five minutes to 15 minutes tops and you get this healthy, delicious, fantastic meal. I'm telling you right now, it's eating right for life, baby.

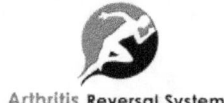

NOTES

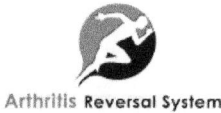

pH

We've got the water. We've got the juicing, blending and fermenting to help heal the gut. Let's look at foods that we can eat that are going to start changing the acidity of our blood. You have to look at if you're taking in acid forming foods.

Remember this is no refined foods. This is no packaged foods if you can get away with that. I know some people that live in extreme environments; you're going to have to eat some type of preserved food. It's hard to get fresh vegetables in northern Canada in January, I totally understand that. You can get the fermented, you can get the canned, but try and make sure that those cans are organic vegetables inside of the cans and make sure the lining of the can . . . know it's tough. In our country, in America, we line the can with BPA, which is a toxic plastic which leeches into the food and makes the healthy plants inside toxic.

Make sure the foods that you're getting are organic if possible, 70 percent plant based which would be ideal and now let's go over sample breakfast lunches and dinners.

BREAKFAST

Liter of water first. A healthy breakfast would be say a bowl of oatmeal, with oatmeal, make sure that it's going to be organic and you can mix honey in there. You can even have coffee *with sugar*.

You're saying wait a second. He's recommending coffee? Yes. Coffee does have a lot of benefits in gastric motility. However, the reason I say you have to have a little bit of natural sugar, and this could be maple syrup, honey or raw sugar. When that caffeine hits your blood, it increases the metabolic response. It increases your energy. You start going crazy.

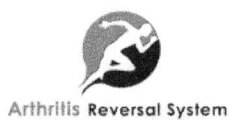

If you have a simple carbohydrate in that drink and that's what that sugar is, your body has something that it can burn. If it has that sugar in there, it can start burning and utilize the caffeine then the caffeine or the coffee or tea won't have a negative effect on the adrenal glands and that's vital.

You live your life through your nervous system and I got to tell you, I keep going back to the thyroid function, we're talking about healthy joints, healthy diet, you've got to look at the adrenals when you're talking about a healthy diet and healthy nutrition.

Now, so coffee with sugar is okay, but make sure that it's organic coffee. They use a tremendous amount of pesticides in the coffee industry, so make sure it's harvested correctly, make sure it's organic coffee. That's something that you can do.

Also, and it may seem like a lot of work, but you're worth it. Remember, anything you put in your body becomes you. Do not buy the fresh ground beans. Get a coffee grinder and grind it yourself. The reason is, the rich oils, the oils inside of the coffee that actually have benefit but go bad pretty quickly. They turn rancid and it also loses some of its antioxidant capabilities. I recommend that you get a coffee grinder and you grind it fresh, each cup or each pot.

20 cups of coffee a day will kill you. We recommend you've got to get five or less cups of coffee a day. That will be ideal and for goodness sake, don't take it right before bed, because that's going to give you a stimulant and you're not going to be able to experience deep sleep.

Good breakfast. Fresh bowl of oatmeal. You could put some fruit on there. You could put some honey on there. It's just absolutely fantastic. If you want to, you could even put some coconut milk. There's certain things that you can drink with a meal.

Dairy

Dairy products. A lot of people nowadays are lactose intolerant, but that's not really true. They're lactose intolerant because the milk products that we have in this country are extremely toxic. A cow, just like a goat and just like a sheep and just like a buffalo and just like a human only gives milk during or after they're pregnant. They get pregnant, they start to lactate and the milk comes out.

In this country, we give them a tremendous amount of hormones to keep them pregnant and producing milk all the time. A dairy cow should live about 20 or 25 years. In this country, they die off after about four or five years because we just deplete their body of everything and so then the milk becomes toxic. It has antibiotics. It has hormones in it. It's really a sick, sick product.

If you're going to drink dairy, make sure it's from a healthy cow, grass fed, no antibiotics, no hormones and then you have to look for pasteurization and homogenization. Homogenization is how you take a healthy dairy product and turn it into a toxic dairy product. They actually take these big, large, fat globules inside of the milk that your body can utilize and they blast it into a stainless steel plate so that the fat is diffused throughout the milk and so now, in modern times and I'm talking just about the last 40 to 50 years, people are used to seeing a glass of milk that's one color. It's all homogenized fat. In the old days, or if you're getting raw milk or non-homogenized milk, the cream literally floats to the top so it has two different colors in there.

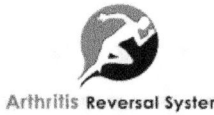

That type of milk is going to be beneficial. For a lot of people, if you're not lactose intolerant, it's actually beneficial for the thyroid. It actually gives you healthy fats in order to regenerate a fat soluble vitamins, because you do need carbohydrates, proteins and fats and milk is actually a pretty good source of it if it's from a healthy animal, but it can be a main stay to your diet.

You're not going to have a gallon of milk a day or tons and tons of cheese, because that's a terrific amount of fat. In certain climates on our planet, the dairy is actually one of the healthier sources of a high energy food called fat because fat is just stored energy. If you're in the colder climates, you may require that.

We've got no water 20 minutes before a meal, no water during, no water after. Oatmeal with fresh fruit and either coconut milk, almond milk or regular milk, but make sure it's healthy from grass fed non-homogenized, non-pasteurized.

If you can also, get fresh fruit. You get fresh fruit in the morning, that's a simple carbohydrate and that's in the morning when your body starts to increase its energy, so you need fast burning nutrients in the morning. Fresh fruit is also a fantastic breakfast.

There's also fresh fruit and yogurt and if you're a vegan, you can get coconut yogurt. You can get a lot of different cultures and the benefit of yogurt whether it's from a cow, buffalo or sheep or a coconut, okay because that's actually one of my favorite yogurts, mix some fresh fruit and some walnuts in there. Then you're going to get healthy omega3s, healthy bacteria.

NOTES

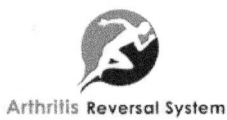

LUNCH

Then this takes you through breakfast. Then let's go into lunch. When you're eating lunch, what I want you to do and this is tough to get this concept. I want you to *eat when you're hungry*. Not on schedule.

How many times have you been in an office setting?

"Yeah, I'm not really hungry."
"Let's go to lunch."
"OK."

No!
You eat when you're hungry. Your body is intelligent. It's going to tell you when you need more nutrients.

What I want you to avoid though is to eat for pleasure. Living to eat they say, or to eat when you're nervous or eat when you're upset. You don't need to eat lunch. If you choose to, or if you're hungry, fantastic. Make sure it's 70 percent plant at least.

70 percent raw plant would be ideal because remember your body is 70 percent water. Fresh vegetable juice for lunch, raw plants or vegetables, salads are fantastic and what you can do, if you don't like just straight salads, let's get creative. Put some jicama root in there. Put some walnuts. Put some dried fruits in there. You can't imagine how good a salad can be when you sprinkle some pine nuts on there.

Get these flavors and then also let's use some spices in there as well. Let's use a little bit of sea salt. Let's use a little bit of black pepper which helps with digestion. Let's use cayenne pepper. Mix it all in there and if you like, even lightly sauté it. Sauté it in

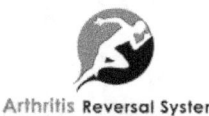

coconut oil and that right there, if you sauté broccoli, you sauté carrots, you sauté some root vegetables, you can actually release more of the nutrients inside of them. This is why we recommend juicing so much.

Get creative and I know there's a lot of people saying well, what about the protein? Hey, you get more protein in spinach then you do in most burgers from McDonald's and hopefully you're just driving by those McDonald's. That's not a healthy food.

Start looking at the nutrients you put in your system. Now, you make it through. What kind of snacks are you going to have during the day? Well, I got to tell you. Raw chocolate is one of the best. Super high in minerals, but you got to look at the label.

When I say 100 percent dark chocolate, raw chocolate, all of these things, it's going to taste really bitter and so what we want to do, since chocolate is such a fantastic energy food, fantastic mineral replacement, take it and dip it in some local honey. That right there my friends is the best afternoon snack you're ever going to have.

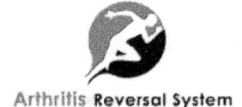

NOTES

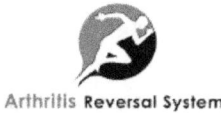

DINNER

Let's go on through dinner. Dinner, you want to make sure you're not eating two hours before your bedtime. Dinner is going to be essential, but you can't eat too late. With my schedule it's kind of tough, because I work until about 8:30, 9:00. I always try and have a snack before I go into my late night health talks or my second or third shift.

I understand that some people get home 8:00, 9:00. Hey, I get up at 4:00. That doesn't leave a heck of a lot of time. Make sure that you think about what you're eating the next day. Prepare your meals in advance. When you heat up food, and this is why it's really tough to have a raw lifestyle or a raw vegan lifestyle, because when you heat food up, it releases these beautiful molecules and they hit the inside of your nose. You've got a piece of your brain exposed called the olfactory bulb and this is how you smell. Let's look for healthy dinner starches.

RESTRICTIONS

There's certain restrictions. If you are getting over cancer or if you're recovering from certain thyroid disorders, you don't want to have raw greens, raw kale or raw spinach or raw cruciferous vegetables. You need to have those cooked or sautéed slightly. If you're eating beans, those have an inhibitory enzyme in there.

Normal, healthy people can tolerate this food and not just tolerate it, we can thrive off it. In fact, dark and leafy vegetables are so loaded with nutrients, as long as you don't have a thyroid issue, you could eat it raw, you could eat it sautéed and the reason I say sautéed is because you don't want to overcook it. You want to cook it just slightly so this allows those excitatory molecules, those molecules to break off of the thick plants, it hits your brain and that stimulates digestion.

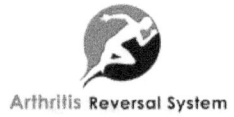

Healthy starches are okay. Healthy wild rice, healthy potatoes and you'll see again, I've got a number of recipes called one pot wonders where you're boiling the potatoes on top of the potatoes, you're steaming some jalapenos. You're steaming some tomatoes. You're steaming some spinach and then you take the slightly steamed vegetables off and mash up the potatoes, put a little bit of coconut oil and mix in all the vegetables. I'm telling you right now, that is a great meal.

I'll make that meal the day before, because sometimes you can't eat after 8:00 at night if you're going to bed at 9:00 or 10:00. You have to eat about three to four hours before you go to bed and make sure that you're not getting simple carbohydrates right before bed.

Ideally if you've had trouble sleeping and I know I'm taking a long time on this one, but you've got to initiate sleep. Sleep is when your body regenerates. That's when the parasympathetic nervous system, which is called rest, digest and repair mode kicks in.

If you're having trouble sleeping, then take in a little bit of protein in your system and this doesn't mean a hunk of chicken or a slice of beef. You can take in some sautéed spinach. Sautéed spinach with a little bit of garlic and a little turmeric. What does that do? It fights cancer, it's an anti-microbial. It's 28 percent protein and you get this in that little snack at night, I'm going to tell you this is fantastic.

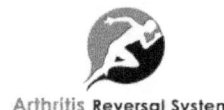

NOTES

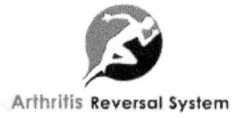

SUMMARY

That's going to take you through sample breakfasts', lunches and dinners. Now, I know it's tough, particularly if you're used to going to restaurants. I know it's tough if you're not cooking.

To reverse disease, to regenerate your tissue, to allow your blood to be healthy, to get those joints to regenerate meniscus and cartilage, you absolutely have to watch what you're putting into your system. Does that make sense?

Organic if possible, 70 to 80 percent of your diet either lightly sautéed or raw, 70 to 80 percent of your meals have to contain fluid. If you're going to eat animals once a month and once a year is great. If you're going to eat it and you're used to having animal products every day, once a week. I'm not asking for much, but a plant based diet. It's better for the planet, it's better for your body, it's better for your system and then to heal digestive issues and you've got to heal the gut first. You've got to get your nervous system checked because that initiates it.

Remember I say when you smell that broccoli that hits the brain, the brain sends a signal down to the stomach? If there's a loss of connection or distorted connection, you're not going to produce the appropriate nutrients or you're not going to produce the appropriate acids to break it down, so you have to get your nervous system checked primarily.

You have to heal the gut. If you've had gut issues for years, you can start healing it. It takes about 30 days. Go to fermented foods, go to juicing or blending. That pre-digests the food and you have to go with a plant-based diet and then once the gut's healed, then you start slowly introducing it.

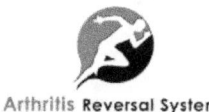

Just change one meal a day. Just one a day. Do that for a couple of weeks. Then you change two meals a day. Do that for a couple of weeks.

I don't want you to take away anything. I want you to add stuff. I want you to add more healthy foods. Even if, let's say you smoke cigarettes, make sure it's organic tobacco. Make sure you eat a piece of fresh fruit with every cigarette. I know that sounds crazy. I had a patient who was smoking three packs of cigarettes a day. That's an addiction, baby, but it also gives them pleasure and joy.

I said great, go out there and hand roll them, so he had that tactile sensation, that tactile stimulus and he went from three packs a day down to less than ten cigarettes a day because it took him so long and he wasn't missing anything. And then I said okay, now what we want to do, we want to add a piece of fresh fruit every time you smoke a cigarette.

Can you see this? Three packs a day, super acidic body, joint pain everywhere, down to ten cigarettes a day and then he was down to five cigarettes a day because he could only eat five pieces of fresh fruit a day. Cool, huh? I'm the only doctor to get him off of that stuff. Why? I just taught him. I taught him little, tiny tricks.

Do these little diet changes. I want you to keep a record. You got to keep a record of what you're doing, because honestly, if you're not drinking that water, if you're looking at the meals, start writing down what you're eating during the day. Keep a journal just for one week. Find out how much fast food you're taking in, how much bread products, how much healthy foods, how much animal products, how much preserved products.

We have all the charts in our ACTION MANUAL and you're going to be able to list all of that. The calorie count I'm not

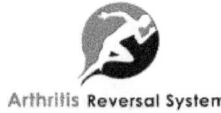

focusing in on as much as the quality count. The quality of what you put in your body is the quality of life you're going to have. The reason we pray over our meals is one, to thank our creator for giving us the food. The other is this is the spiritual aspect. This food becomes you. Choose wisely my friends, okay? You're going to eat for health. God bless.

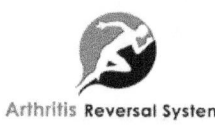

NOTES

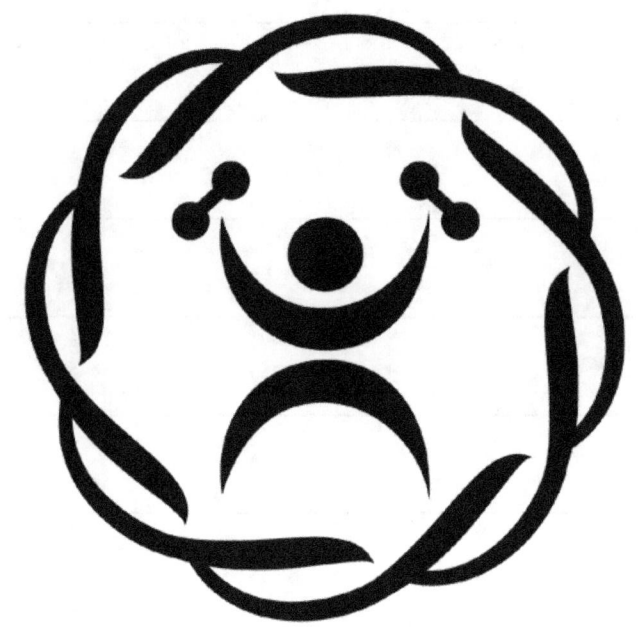

REGENERATIVE EXERCISES

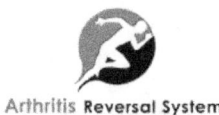

EXERCISE

Exercise for healthy joints. Now this is the most, I wouldn't say the most important, but if you don't move it you lose it, guaranteed. Okay, now this is going to be not just vital, but we're going to go over anatomy, physiology, neurology, and position of the joints in a half hour or less, so hopefully you're watching this in a chair with a seatbelt, because we're going to get wild.

Now movement; remember two bones coming together surrounded by a joint capsule. What we need to do is regenerate those structures inside. We're talking about healthy joints.

MUSCLE TYPES

Now there are three types of muscle in the human body; smooth muscle, cardiac muscle, and skeletal muscle. Smooth muscle, that's the organ systems basically. That rarely gets tired, it can keep functioning forever. If smooth muscle does get tired it can replenish and relax in about 30 seconds.

The heart muscle is amazing. This heart starts beating at about five weeks and keeps going for the next 120 years. That heart never gets tired.

Now let's talk about skeletal muscle. This is the most important muscle group when we're talking about regenerating joints.

Remember, two bones coming together, those bones have either cartilage or meniscus on the inside of it, and that's surrounded by a joint capsule. Now in order to move it, it has to move correctly, because if you have a joint that's misaligned it's not going to function correctly. So we have to look at muscle balance.

Now if you've ever seen somebody with a pulled hamstring; these are professional athletes, athletes that just train and train, so they have muscle memory. Does a pulled hamstring happen quickly or slowly? I've got to tell you, if you've ever seen it, it's like someone shot that person in the back of the leg. So we've got to look at not just the joints, we have to look at the muscles that surround that joint for appropriate motion.

Inside of that joint capsule there are joint mechanoreceptors, and these are sensors that tell your body whether the limb is straight or bent, and it fires off the muscles. So when you take an arm and you bend it instantly on bending it this muscle here contracts, this one instantly relaxes. When you straighten it this one relaxes and this one contracts. So you have that contracting relaxing contracting relaxing, and you have to have that healthy nerve supply to the joint in order to have it function correctly.

You'll see some of our videos; I demonstrate patellar tracking, because you've got the knee joint that has these two bones that come together and it doesn't work like hinge; it works more like a screw where it moves twice as much on the inside as it does on the outside. But it also, there's a patella in there, that knee cap; there are muscles that guide the action of that knee cap. So if the muscles are firing incorrectly, or one is stronger than the other, and

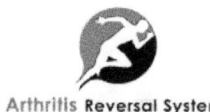

that's called incorrect patellar tracking, you're never going to heal the knee unless you get that corrected.

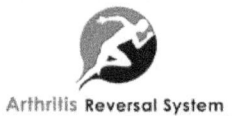

Watch the series of videos on joint regenerative exercises by scanning the QR code below or going to the URL below.

http://0s4.com/r/LHOZK0

Now also when we look at every joint, you've heard of carpel tunnel syndrome, you've heard of tennis elbow, golfer's elbow, shoulder, rotator cup problems. How many people have joint pain in their hand? Well, we have to start with a healthy nerve supply, and those nerves that originate in the spine, the signals go from the brain down the spinal cord and out to supply it. So you have to get your nervous system checked before we start exercising. And you have to understand how the muscles function, and we're going to go over that a bit, too. So you have to get your nervous system checked; that's primary, A-1, number one.

NOTES

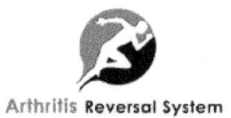

Muscle Imbalances

Then you have to check muscle balance of the joints, and there are several methods to do that, but hopefully a qualified corrective chiropractor will be able to lead you through that.

And also we have to look at strength ratio. If you just take the full arm, normal strength ratio should be five to four. These muscles are called flexors; these are called extensors, and that means that they should be about the same strength; however, in modern society if your job entails you to just grab and grab and move things your flexors are going to be a lot stronger than the extensors. And what that does is that creates a muscle imbalance, and that muscle imbalance is going to negatively affect the elbow joint. And if that muscle imbalance of the forearm, it's also going to negatively affect the wrist. And that muscle imbalance of the forearm is going to negatively affect the elbow, the wrist, and the shoulder. This is why carpel tunnel syndrome, rotator cuff problems, golfer's elbow, tennis elbow, they are all double crush injuries, they all begin with the nerve supply that comes down.

So before we start exercising our arms you have to make sure that you're correcting the problem in the neck. Before we start exercising our legs and how we can build our feet to where they're coiled springs, we have to check the nerve supply in the low back and see if the pelvis is stable; because your foot, you're talking 26 bones, four arches, flexes, bends, turns and twists, and if I hear one more person saying, oh yeah, I have to wear orthotics; my foot is flattening out. No, feet don't flatten out, unless the arches of the foot are a problem, and then on the bottom of the foot you have this fascia called plantar fascia, and if the foot flattens out that inflames.

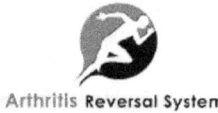

So how many people do you know that say, oh, I've got plantar fasciitis. No you don't; you've got weak intrinsic muscles of the foot. The muscles inside of the foot that operate the foot, not the muscles outside of the foot, okay; so we restore this. And where do the nerves... What's the primary cause of that? It's the nerves that come out of the low back that are actually damaging that, causing a weakness and that causes an altered gait.

This is why checking the nervous system before you exercise is so vitally important. Because every exercise is going to be walking, running, jumping, doing a bounce technique; you're going to be using your arms and legs during exercises.

If you're wheelchair bound we've got to check your neck. Okay, because we're going to be doing a lot of different exercises in order to open and close the joints. So nervous system is number one.

And if you have chronic flat feet, foot problems, bunions; bunions can go away. Check out our video on foot health.

http://0s4.com/r/WAF3RB

When you start looking at swollen joints, joints are alive. As long as you can bend it you can regenerate it. If you've got a joint that's fused we're going to work around it, we're going to do whatever we can; so healthy nerve supply first.

NOTES

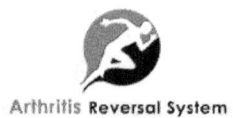

Anatomy

Now let's look at the muscles. A muscle goes across a joint, and it attaches via a tendon. Now that tendon attaches on a connection point, so that means around every joint there's no muscles crossing those joints, there's just tendons. Now every time you open and close a joint, every time you open and close this joint that muscle is contracting and expanding. So those tendons are wrapping and stretching across the joint.

Now the reason, because you can just rub your hands like this and you can feel the temperature start to increase; that's because friction actually increases temperature. So the way you're designed, every tendon is surrounded by a capsule called a sac, a bursa sac. Now those tendons, see, every muscle attaches to the bone via a tendon, and if I hear one more time somebody say, I have bursitis. Think of this; you've got those tendons that cross the joint; they are covered by a sac, and that's filled with bursa fluid. That sac is called the bursa sac and -itis means inflammation.

So all of these people that say, oh, I have bursitis; I have this bursitis, I have that bursitis, and they take a medication for it, but that's really counter-productive. Okay? You figure bursitis of the shoulder, the elbow or the wrist is going to come from the head being too far forward. What that does is choke the blood supply off and it can also affect the nerve supply, so it's almost like your arm is starving for blood. It's like you have a tourniquet on it and you can't get the healthy blood supply to it.

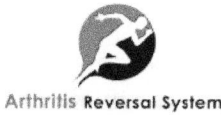

MOIST HEAT

So what we've got to do is we've got to take that tourniquet off before we start exercising and reposition the head. Does that mean that we've got to fix forward head carriage before we start? No, what I want you to do is, we need to find out the source of it. You never want to take a drug for bursitis, and this is how you treat bursitis. Okay, if you have it, or instead of saying bursitis, let's call it what it really is; how to treat lack of fluid to the joint. Ah, that makes more sense. That's where moist heat gets on, because you know the moist heat gets in there, the wetter the better, the deeper the penetration. That moist heat gets on that joint and it fills up that bursa sac with fluid and then you can start working the joint.

Okay, so make sure if you have bursitis anywhere, and this can be in the knees, the patella, the hips, the feet, the ankles, anything; find out what's causing the blood supply problem and then you can override that by putting moist heat on it. And why? Just think what moist heat does. You've got a joint that's drying up, it's desiccating. That joint doesn't have enough fluid, so when you put heat on there and you take it off what color is the skin? It's red. Okay, and the reason it's red is because you're body is increasing the blood pressure to that area to equalize the temperature.

So we're kind of playing a trick on the body here. So even if you have forward head carriage or muscle imbalances, or toxic blood that's causing that bursa sac to inflame then we can override that by changing the temperature that causes more blood supply to flow to it, that fills up the bursa sac, and then that bursa sac takes the pressure off of the joint. Does that make sense? I know it does. We're just listening to the body.

NOTES

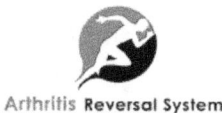

Golgi Tendon Organ

So now you've got the skeletal muscle attaching to the bone, and there's also an organ inside of that tendon. I mean it sounds crazy, but you do, it's called a Golgi tendon organ, a GTO. I know, just like the car, baby. Okay now, these things govern the strength of the muscle, and I'm going to show you how to reset those as well.

So, healthy nerve supply before we start exercising. Let's regenerate or check the joint mechanoreceptors, and the muscles surrounding the joints. Okay, and then we can start exercising. And the ideal exercise is to start moving. See, when you take a joint and you open and close it, that allows or creates a negative pressure and a positive pressure, and this is just somebody walking. They're just walking along and they're creating a negative pressure and a positive pressure. And that causes a pumping action on the joints. So move every joint every day, at least a couple of times. That's going to be the best exercise to regenerate it.

Now the discs of the spine; they have a horrible blood supply. Even the way the knee works, the plateau, because you've got one bone down here that's the tibia; you've got the femur that comes on top, and a lot of people say, well, the meniscus can't regenerate because there's no blood supply to it. No, the body's smarter than that. If that femur is resting on top and you're whole weight is standing on that that's hundreds of pounds of pressure; blood vessels would be crushed. So the meniscus of the knee, and that's the covering that holds that knee joint in place, that guides it. It's kind of like a thick Tupperware where it guides the joint; that outside edge of the meniscus does have a blood supply. The inside of the meniscus doesn't; it gets its nutrients from the synovial fluid. So you don't have dead cells in the body.

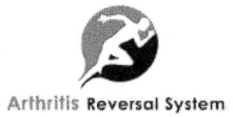

NSAIDs

And I know this is a tough concept because a lot of people have been told, well, now joints just don't re-grow. No kidding. I know most doctors don't re-grow them because they're primary line of therapy is going to be non-steroidal anti-inflammatory drugs, and that's going to be the Motrin, Aleve, Ibuprofen, all of those crazy ones. And Tylenol is not a non-steroidal anti-inflammatory, but even that limits the building blocks of cartilage. So you don't ever want to treat joint pain with a drug that destroys the joints; that's pretty illogical.

Now we know that healthy food creates healthy blood which creates healthy synovial fluid. And a lot of people will say, oh, I can feel the weather's going to change, my joints are starting to ache. Now let's talk about that.

There is pressure inside of that synovial sack. You've got the two bones covered by that sac. There's an electrical sensor in that sac that we have to change, so we have to correct the spinal nerve supply to that. There's a muscle balance that has to be corrected. And that's a balance of the calf, it's a balance of the quadriceps, it's a balance of hamstrings in the quadriceps, it's a balance of the extensors and flexors of the muscles. It's a balance of the agonist and antagonist muscles. So we need to have healthy balance.

And if you do repetitive tasks at one job or you've done activities on a regular basis or you're a one-sided sport person, you have to train to build the muscles that you don't use during the day. So have your corrective chiropractor check your body thoroughly to find the muscle imbalances to make sure that the nerve supply is working and then we can start exercising. Okay, does that make sense?

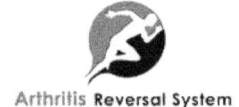

NOTES

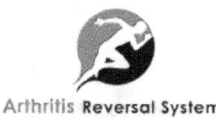

Start Where You Are

Now if you do have joint pain I don't want you to work on something... I don't want you to walk on arthritic knees, I don't want you running on damaged flat feet, I don't want you doing crazy yoga positions where you're sucking your toe and putting it behind your head. Let's start where we can.

If all you can do is sit, great. What I want you to do is, and this is one of the exercises that we recommend, is you put a water bottle behind your back, right about the level of the bottom of the ribcage. Put it back there for 20 minutes, take it out for 10, back there for 20 minutes, take it out for ten. What that does is it causes the pelvis to rock. If you have a sedentary job get a ball chair; the ball chairs are fantastic because you're always sitting on an uneven surface.

One of the most brilliant chiropractors and physiologists of our time, Dr. James Chestnut, says we have no genetic defense against sitting. Sitting is absolutely devastating to the structures of the spine. So if you do sit, and this is going to do with the exercises for the entire lower extremities; if you were to golf, say, eight hours a day and you said, wow, my back is sore. No kidding. When you golf, that golf swing, the pressure on the L5-S1 disc; this is the disc right at the base, increases eight times normal. When you sit it increases five times normal.

So we're talking that if you're sitting for five to six hours a day you're damaging those discs. And guess what; the L5-S1 disc, you've got to figure, is so important because when we're talking about foot problems, plantar fasciitis, we're talking bunions, we're talking all the foot ailments, we're talking knee problems. It all stems from improper mechanics and pinched nerve supply. So remember, if you're golfing the pressure on that disc increases eight times.

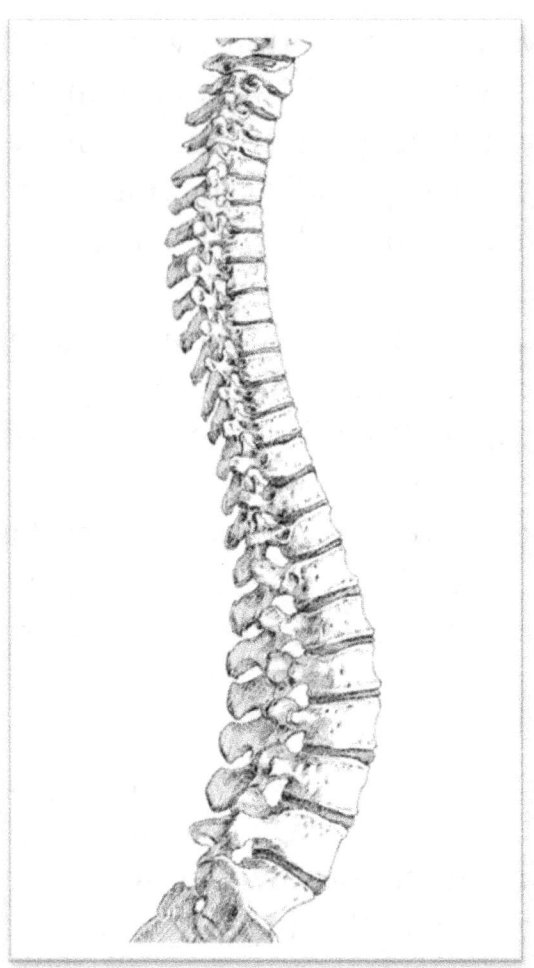

Okay, so when we look at this, this is the side view of a human body. Here's the head up here, and you should normally have beautiful, beautiful curves from the side. From the front it should be straight up and down. Now we're talking about this disc right here. When you sit, you sit on this bone here. It flattens out the curve in the lower back and that actually reverses the discs. But it opens up the holes where the nerves come out. So sitting feels good; however, you're reversing the discs. And if this remains this way you're going to be bent over in a chronic bent position and

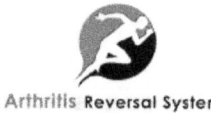

this is not a sign of age, but it's a sign of disc damage and dehydration.

So if you see someone walking bent over, they're trying to adapt to a toxic deficient circumstance. Well, these discs are alive; if you can move them, you can regenerate them. You can re-grow them; they're living tissue. But you've got to figure, every time since these discs are under such huge compressive force loads, they have a horrible blood supply. They get their nutrients through movement, and that's what we're going to talk about. See, exercise is only healthy nerve supply, healthy muscle balance, healthy blood supply, and movement. I know, it seems too simple, because it is.

CONSULT A CORRECTIVE CHIROPRACTOR

Now I'm going to show you the greatest exercise to start your day with, and this is something that we go in and again, *you've got to get to a corrective chiropractor first*. Because I'm going to show you some exercises that may be appropriate for you or may not be.

If we typically get patients with disc injuries of this area, this area or this area, this is one of the more common areas; the low back and the neck are, for disc injuries. So usually it takes me about two to three weeks before I can have them do this twisting exercise, and this is the greatest one.

So this exercise involves movement, and usually we get people who have had severe disc injuries, and they can do this in about two to three weeks after we get some adjustments in there.

What I want you to do is you're going to stand with your hands out away from your body. Now the reason your hands are like this is for momentum. See, this right here probably weighs maybe 10 or 15 pounds, so I've got two of them. So for momentum it's like taking a sledge hammer and swinging it around your body; you're going to be able to move beyond the normal range of motion.

And this is what I want to explain to you. Normal range of motion, and range of motion has to do with everything; this is as far as I can bend my finger in a normal range of motion. Okay? And that's called active. Passive range of motion is much further, where I can bend it even further than that. What we want to do is move you in what's called the paraphysiologic range of motion. But we only want to be there for a fraction of a second; that's even further than passive. And you can do this to regenerate the joints.

Now if you are not used to exercising, let's say that you can only turn your head this far or that far, that's because you haven't been moving it. So what we want to do is work those joints. Now any time you do an exercise, anytime you do a therapy, if you're my patient any time I tell you to do something if you're sore more than an hour you're pushing it too hard. If you're sore less than an hour you probably could go a little bit harder. Because we're taking joints that haven't moved correctly or degenerated or are toxic, and toxic bodies, and we're going to re-grow that joint, regenerate the joint and regenerate movement.

So this is one of the greatest exercises ever. You're hands are like this, away from your body, and you throw them. And I want you to turn from the hips all the way up; you don't need to turn the knees, just from the hips all the way up. And you're going to turn as far as you can. And what I want you to do is head, neck, everything, as far as you can so you're looking almost behind you. But I want you to do it quickly, because remember, we're trying to get to that paraphysiologic range of motion, that range of motion that's beyond active.

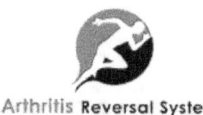

Okay, and turn this way as far as you can; again, head, neck, everything turns as far as you can. But what I want you to do now, and this is the scary part, I want you to do it quickly. So back and forth, as quickly as you can. And what that does, if you do 100 of them, and you could break it up, 25 four times a day. I start and finish my workout with it, but also what I want you to do is if you have a balance issue, like let's say you've been doing medications for years, or let's say you're dehydrated. That twisting may cause you to be not stable, so I want you to lean up against, say, a washing machine, or a table or chair so you can have a little bit more stability.

If you're wheelchair bound do it in a chair. Okay, I mean, if your balance is horrible, like let's say you've been taking cholesterol and blood pressure drugs, which is just completely toxic, you're going to have major balance issues. This is why a lot of blood pressure drugs are actually associated with falls, because if you don't have enough blood to the brain your body is going to kick the legs out from underneath you to get your head level to get more oxygen up to it. So a lot of people are taking medications and they're falling. So do that only if you have a healthy balance, and if you can't do it standing up, do it sitting down. We just want to move those joints to get them healthy.

Safe Lifting

Now when you're exercising, and this is super important, when you're exercising and you'll see a lot of people do this in gym; they'll take a great weight and they'll start here and they'll lift up as high as they can, and then they'll go back down. Okay, that is so dangerous for unhealthy joints. It looks good, but you don't want to do that to regenerate the joints. You never want to have a joint that's at its extreme end range of motion, and then put it under a strain.

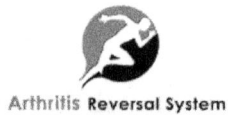

What we want to do since we're working with joints and we want to get them healthy, this is how you're going to exercise. Have a weight where your joint, and I'm demonstrating the shoulder joint now. It's not going to be here where it's unstable; it's going to be right here, and all I want you to do is move it just about five or six inches up, five or six inches back down. If you're doing curls where you're bending the bicep like this, you don't want to start with the arm extremely strained. You want to start with it bent already to 90 degrees, and then you want to go up just slightly, and then down.

And now we've got to talk about it, and this is the secret. Concentric and eccentric contractions; okay, now you've got to know this anatomy since you're alive in a human body. Muscle fibers can only do two things; they can contract, which means they get shorter, or they can elongate. Okay, this is a concentric contraction; this is an eccentric contraction. This is a secret, you build more muscle on eccentric contractions. That means if you can lower the weight slowly you're going to build more muscle. You build more muscle, you get more mass, you get more mass; your body mass index gets healthier. And you can actually burn more calories, too.

So what we want, you never want to work a joint full range of motion when it's under stress. Full range of motion should be used for Pilates or used for yoga to where you can allow your joints to move fully, allow them to open and close; that's going to be essential. When we're talking about resistance exercises you want to do very heavy weights, very short range of motions, and you want to go slowly. You'll see too many people in the gym where they throw the weight up and they throw the weight up, it looks impressive, but you can't do that with unhealthy joints, and it's not really effective or efficient.

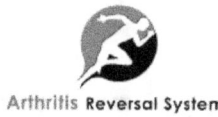

So what you want is a very heavy weight, moved very slowly. And this heavy weight for someone in their 80's that's never exercised could be two pounds. Okay, so experiment around, start light and work your way up. But now you're only going to do this any kind of resistance exercise about four to five reps. And so what it's going to look like if you're working biceps you have a weight here.

So you've got a seven and a half pound ankle weight, or hand weight. No, just one is good. My genie that throws stuff was trying to get two aggressive. So when you do this what I want you to do is you're going to lift it up, but take about 15 seconds to lift it up, and take about 15 seconds to lower it down.

But I want you to breathe. See, if you're not oxygenating your system then your body is going to start to produce more lactic acid. Now lactic acid is not bad; in fact lactic acid actually increases the firing and increases your endurance, so it's actually beneficial. But if you're producing too much lactic acid that means you're not breathing during that exercise. So when you're doing those weight exercises it's [breathing] and then keep breathing on the way down. You're hyper-oxygenating. Every time you take a breath you're also helping to move lymph, and you can start with very light weight to where you get your range of motion.

NOTES

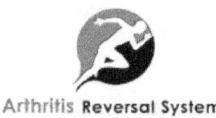

Range of Motion

So range of motion should only be very limited if you're doing resistance, and to open and close we really recommend stretches, yoga, and you'll see a number of diagrams in the back of our exercise book that's going to show you how to slowly work into this. You've got to get the healthy nerve supply, you've got to get the muscle balance, because I've got to tell you, if you have a long-term low back problem and you have imbalance of the quadriceps, the muscles of the knee, then bike riding is not going to be good for you; walking is not going to be good for you. If you have flattening of the feet and I tell you to start getting on a jumper, that's not going to work either. You absolutely need to get your nervous system corrected; your blood supply corrected, and then start exercising a half hour a day to sweat.

I know it sounds crazy, but a half hour, 30 minutes a day to where you're working hard enough to where you sweat, and start a little at a time. If you're going to a store, park far away; park a couple of blocks away from your work and walk to lunch, or walk to breakfast, or walk to the market; start walking a bit more if you can, just a little bit at a time. I do talks in Chicago in the wintertime and I'm walking on the street, and I'm telling you right now, baby, that's cold. It's cold outside. But you've still got to walk. Okay, walking is the best exercise you can have.

And then let's say you have osteoporosis, or you've had a very acidic condition. There's a small trampoline called a rebounder, and you can start just by bouncing on that rebounder and that's going to be an excellent exercise. That's going to strengthen the bone, it's going to move the lymph, and just that small bouncing up actually allows the fluid to flow, and it gets your muscles working.

So resistance exercises, you have to do at least three or four days a week if not every day; make sure it's short range of motion, make sure you do them slow, heavy weight contractions up, and heavy weight contractions down. How many should you do? I want you to do it to fatigue, to where you just can't lift it up anymore. And that should be about four to five. So this way you're working the muscle, but you're not working the joint.

Now all of these exercises are going to be demonstrated, okay. The turning exercises, the twisting exercises, but heal the joints and get the joints healthy first. And it should be done in conjunction, you know, don't wait. If you have very arthritic joints, don't wait to start the exercise program; it has to be in harmony with the medication reduction, with the diet and nutrition changes, and the healthier nerve supply. Even if you're just seeing this tape, start slow. If it hurts to move a joint, put moist heat on it. And then if you can move it more then you know that it's just from lack of fluid in the joint where the joint pain is coming from. Get the healthy nutrients.

NOTES

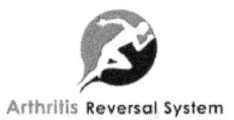

Can I Tell You a Secret?

And now I'm going to tell you another secret. After your workout you're going to be depleted of electrolytes. You're going to need some healthy nutrients. So get coconut water; coconut water is one of the greatest fast electrolyte replacements that you're going to have, and then this way you're not too sore. You can also have a hot shower, a hot bath after the workout; that's going to help stimulate the lymph flow, and if you can do a contrast bath where it's very hot to very cold, very hot to very cold, that absolutely eliminates any build up of the lactic acid and you're going to feel not just refreshed, but your health is going to be much, much better. But have your corrective chiropractor direct what exercises are appropriate for your body.

And in the Action Journal, I want you to mark off each day that you're exercising, each day that you're improving. And also, I want you to mark down, because this is really exciting, if you're doing resistance training, you're going to see your strength improve in just a matter of weeks. If you're going from absolutely no exercising, a hundred pounds over-weight, and everything else, you're going to be amazed at how fast you can regenerate your tissue, regenerate the joints and regenerate your exercise capabilities. So mark that in your Action Journal.

And I've got to tell you, I'm so excited to be involved with you. You're going to love working out. I'll see you at the gym.

NOTES

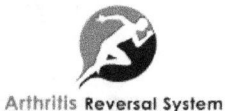

HEALING MINDSET

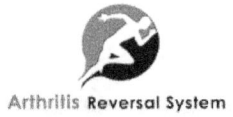

SELF-TALK

Self-talk, changing your perception. This is absolute key when it comes to disease reversal. Since we're focusing in on arthritis with this video series, imagine if you could control your genes. You can. You see, there's an epi-genetic control. Epi- means above, so there's a control above that controls gene expression.

Now, we're talking about arthritis so what does gene expression have to do with tissue regeneration? Everything. I mean, everything. If you change your focus... See we're coming into a world now that we're understanding that the body is more energy than matter. We know this. You're seeing me. I look solid, but I'm actually 70 trillion cells held together with thought. So if you can change your thought, you can change your perception, you can change the outcome.

Now, if you're stuck in a mindset that your body is old or degenerated or it runs in my family. You're never going to heal. You've got to change your perception. If you've been going to the medical system, the sick care system that we have now and they've labeled you with *bam*, some type of diagnosis... you have high cholesterol, fibromyalgia, diabetes, whatever. Whatever their label is, understand that you can change the outcome by changing your physiology and you change your perception of that. And you're going to see multiple, multiple diseases, and I'm talking cancers, brain tumors. These can all be reversed through diet, nutrition, exercise, nerve supply. But nothing happens, nothing happens unless you change your thought patterns.

So this is going to be something, because I'm going to share with you a couple of ideas that you can do to change your thought

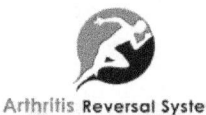

patterns, because a lot of the time our minds get into this negative mindset because it's familiar. If you wake up and you're hurting every day, you're not going to say, oh, I feel great. No, that's lying to yourself. But if you realize that you change your self-talk, that's going to absolutely change the outcome and that's going to stimulate cells.

We want to replace those bad, negative cells in the body. We want to replace the distorted, unhealthy cartilage, the distorted, unhealthy bones. We want to eliminate bone spurs from the body, but it all starts with self-talk and how you change your self-talk. Now, this is going to be new and unfamiliar for a lot of people, but you have to train your brain and train your thought patterns and train your self-talk the same way you train your muscles. We're going for the Olympics of healing, baby.

And this is what we need to start doing. So what I want you to do, if you have a bar of soap. You know how you get out of bed, you shuffle over to the bathroom, you turn the light on, you look in the mirror... what I want you to do is write on that glass "You're perfect just the way you are. You're beautiful, dynamic, you're a health magnet".

NOTES

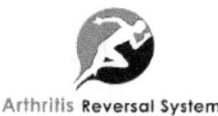

Vision Board

Write something that's going to empower you, but you are perfect just the way you are. We just need to remodel your thought patterns, remodel your diet, remodel your nervous system, and then you have that healthy, dynamic body that attracts wealth, abundance, love, joy, and then you can live your life to your full potential. So, what we're going to do is we're going to start off making a *vision board*. This is going to be very, very important because a lot of people... we get stuck in a mindset that we don't really know what we can do.

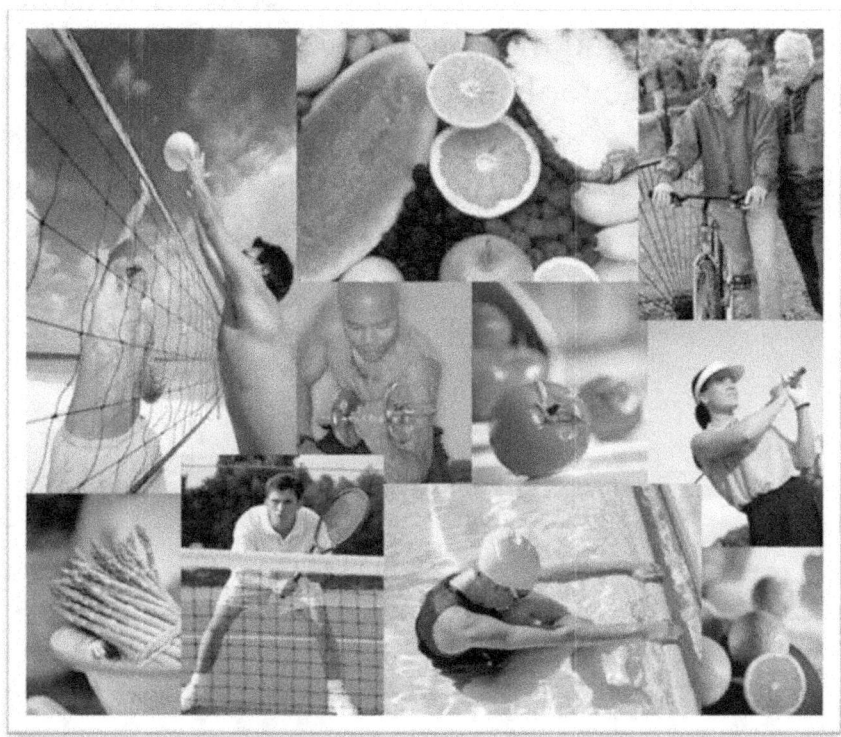

And I have to tell you, it was apparent to me, this was about 35, 40 years ago, I was a contractor. I was working on a kitchen. We were in Chatsworth. Chatsworth, California, it's about 350 degrees in the shade. We were locked in a plastic room because we're remodeling this kitchen. It's demo time and it's dust, sweat is dripping down, I couldn't hardly breathe, but I'm working and ripping and everything else. My buddy next to me, he says, "I can't take this anymore. I'm going swimming." And I went, "You can't go swimming. We have to finish this." And my brain was so stuck in that environment that no matter how torturous or hellacious it was, we had to complete the task even though I was miserable. I was breathing in more toxic dust than a human being should breathe in.

He just changed my mindset. Actually, we went outside, went swimming, came back in. I felt refreshed, I felt renewed, because my mind couldn't look beyond it. It was almost like he was speaking a different language. I couldn't really hear what he was... it didn't make sense. And that's what we have to do with you. I'm going to give you some tools to change your perception.

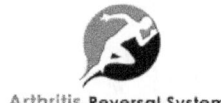

NOTES

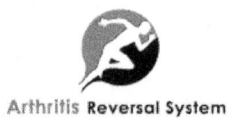

100 Ways to a Better Life

If you think that you're old, if you think you're sick, if you've been labeled with any type of disease we can change that now. And this is not a week-long project. This is something that I want you to do *right now*. I want you to sit down, take out your meditation journal and write 100 things you want to do, be, or become. You want to do, be, or become. One hundred items. Now you could write down ten pretty quick, but remember we're talking about universal intelligence, that there's an intelligence in the body.

There's also intelligence, or universal force that we're all connected to and this is going to help you tap into that because if you just think you're alone, you're single, or you're a dad, or you're a mom, or you're a child and that's who you identify with, I want you to identify with a power greater than yourself. Knowing that you're more energy than matter, and changing that self-talk is actually going to change that perception in your brain to realize that you're greater than yourself.

Your body doesn't stop here. Your influence doesn't stop here. You can see it on photography where there's just energy emanations coming off from your system. I'm going to show you how to tap into that.

Write one hundred things to do, be, or become, and when you get to 20 or 30 or 50 or 60 or 75, you're going to have to come up with some crazy stuff like, walk the Great Wall of China, learn Mandarin, do a cooking class in Tuscany, go on the River Rhine cruise. Come up with anything. Hike to Machu Picchu and no limits. If you're in a wheel chair, if you're degenerated, if you're 100 years old, still you can do anything.

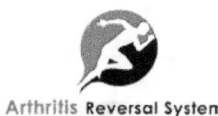

I just read an article about the oldest woman to sail around the woman nonstop. She's 70. I mean, we have no limits. The oldest person to scale Mount Fuji in Japan was 93 years old. She took up mountain climbing at 85. So when I say no limits, I mean no limits.

When, you've got your list of 100 things. Next to that, I want you to put a one, five, or ten next to each one. The things that you're going to accomplish in one year, the things that you're accomplish in five years or less, things that you're going to accomplish in ten years or less. And then, you go through, I know it takes a lot of work but by gosh you're worth it. You have to do this 100 things to do, be, or become at least once a year. January is a great time but by gosh if it's April, start in April. Start now. Don't wait. The fortune favors the bold. Alexander [the Great] was right.

So you write it down, then you pick the top five of the one year, the top five of the five years, and the top five of the ten years, and that's what you're going to make your vision board out of. The vision board is a collection of pictures. If you're good with a computer, great. Just go to Google images, type in the picture you want and put it on there. So if you want a great relationship, put the ideal person on that picture. If you want wealth and abundance, or health, if you want wisdom... and it doesn't have to be living people. On my vision board, I actually put Yoda from Star Wars so it could be anybody. Anybody whose philosophy that you admire.

But make sure that you have this in a place where you can look at it every day. See the whole thing is, many, many people are being programmed by the television, which is okay if you're watching documentaries about life-affirming things. But if you're programming your brain with things like the news or you're being programmed by 56 percent of the advertising on TV which is for drugs, you know, "Ask your doctor if this is right for you", I'm telling you that gets in your psyche. It gets in your personality, and this is what you feel is your body. So you have to do the 100 things to do, be, or become.

Then, you also have to write down on your mirror in the morning "I'm perfect just the way I am".

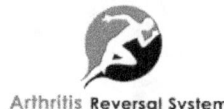

NOTES

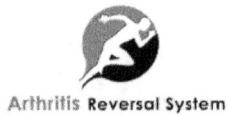

NLP

Then we have to do self-talk. I've done this on hundreds and hundreds of people. It's called neuro-linguistic programming, where you can change your brain by changing the volume, the intonation, the verbiage, and the body language. So we need to change your system in your body. You could have had the worst, most horrific accident. I had this one patient, she was driving down the road in a suburban city, just a suburb. Nice drive and the manhole cover blows up. It lifts her car up off the ground. Do you think that might create a little bit of panic? Yeah.

So with everybody that has chronic illness, they've got the same panic. If every time you move it hurts, you're not going to want to move, so now we need to change our self-talk. Look at how a person stands. If you're standing like the weight of the world is on you, if you're standing like you just had the most darkest moment, you just broke up that relationship you thought was going to last, you had a business problem, more challenges of health, how do you stand? I got to tell you, you're standing like the weight of the world is on you and this is how people are looking. You can see it. When you're people watching in the mall or airport you can see someone that's healthy, dynamic, in charge and some people that are just depressed. They've got the weight of the world on them. And I've got to tell you, when you're standing like you're healthy, in charge, dynamic, bold, excited about life, what's the difference? I'm telling you right now.

Tony Robbins is a master of this, neuro-linguistic programming. I encourage you to check out his videos. The only difference is from depressed and sad to joyous and happy; it's just a couple of millimeters. That's all it is. Even if your brain doesn't accept that you're in a healthy mode. If you're saying my joints are healthy, my joints are healthy, oh gosh, it hurts to lift. That's not going to convince your brain, so I'm talking about reprogramming your brain. You have 100 things to do, be, or become. You've got the words on the mirror, the first thing that you see in the morning. And then I want you to add post-it notes everywhere of positive sayings and life-affirming sayings. Write down some life affirming sayings below to get you started on your journey to health!

_____

_____

_____

_____

_____

_____

_____

_____

_____

_____

_____

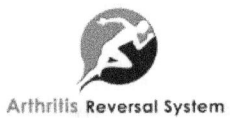

Breathe

So now we're going to do it. You put your body in that posture, your shoulders back, you deep breathe and then I want you to start moving because the brain functions like a battery. To change the brains connection with the body you have to change its input, and the input to the brain requires movement. So this is what I want you to do. I want you to change your brain. Stand up if you can. Put your shoulders back. I want you to deep breathe.

Now when you're happy, how's your tone? Your tone is vital, and the volume is vital because if you're excited you're going to be a little bit louder. And this is a challenge with a lot of my patients that I work with. Some of them are really kind of scared. In fact, if I could have my bear. Sometimes I'm just shy. That's not going to bring joy. Well, how could this not bring joy? But that's different. This is cuddling, but does it feel good? Can it bring you joy? Yes, absolutely.

But when we look at this, look at the different personalities. If you're a personality where you're sad, or depressed, or you just don't get it or you're dynamic, excited, looking forward to life, that's what we want. Change your body posture. Change your body posture to one that's excited.

AFFIRMATIONS

So now we have to do the volume, and I don't want you to go in and just say affirmations. I don't want you to just say oh, I'm healthy, I'm healthy, I'm healthy. The affirmations that you're going to do during this neuro-linguistic programming are going to be present tense. They're going to be right now. Not, I really want

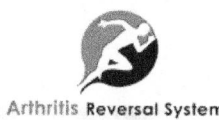

a healthy body. No, that's not going to work. If you're wanting something you are always going to be wanting it. That's what that universe is going to do. It's going to require you to want something your entire life.

So this has got to be present-time consciousness. It's got to be right now, and it's got good volume and you've got to have good motion. Since we are talking about arthritis, "I wish my joints didn't hurt" is not what you're going to say. What you're going to say is, "*my joints are regenerating. I have a strong, healthy, dynamic body. I can feel my joints regrowing. I can feel the meniscus in my knee regenerating. Do you know every time I open and close my joints, blood flows into them. That superfiltrative synovial fluid is constantly being regenerated. My diet is disciplined and effective. I regenerate because I have 80 percent healthy plant foods in my system that's raw. My meals are 70 percent water. I regenerate every day. Every time I move my joint it regrows. I replace a billion cells a day. I am human*".

How could you not... I mean look at this. You do that, and I'm talking just a couple of minutes a day. If you have a financial challenge that's limiting you, then you don't say "I want more money". No. You have to change your perception. "*I live in a world of abundance. Abundance flows to me. I love being financially free*". What about relationships? Do the same thing with relationships. "*I'm connected to my soul mate. She's brilliant, articulate, passionate*". What about relationships with my family? "*I love my family. When we get together, we're one. We're one body. We're one soul. We're one mindset. My sons, myself, we are just so dynamic and when we get together there's magic*".

So it's got to be in present time, but make sure it's dynamic. And I've got to tell you, unless you want to scare the neighbors do it in a car with the windows rolled up. Because honestly, that's how I...

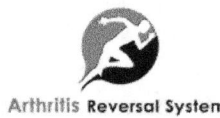

I get up at 4:00 in the morning, I'm adjusting people at 5:00 in the morning. Sundays I work till about 8:30 at night and in order to keep that energy level right when I get to work and maintain it throughout the day, I have to do this. I'm programming my brain for high energy. If you feel like your joints are hurting, if you have any health challenges, change your brain and change your self-talk.

NOTES

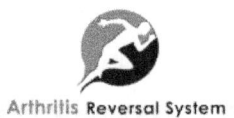

SUMMARY

So you've got the vision board, you've got the 100 things to do, be, or become. Because what could you do if you had no limits? Think of this, we have some exercises we're going to walk you through and I want you to do these mental exercises every day. I want to start programming your brain correctly. You do not program it with the news because the news is wrong. If the news was accurate... I live close to L.A. and Orange County, there's like 17 million people around me. 17 million people and they're focusing in on one traffic accident or one robbery or one this.

Why don't they focus in on the 16 million nine-hundred acts of kindness? Why don't they focus in on how the bag boy at the grocery store carried the groceries out for the senior citizen? How about the people that bring puppies to the assisted living centers. I mean look at this. There are so many acts of kindness that aren't on the news.

You're not getting educated by the news; you're getting programmed by it. So start programming your brain with positive thoughts, with positive images. You can't go in and watch horror movies every night. You know, if you want to great, for fun, but you can't program your brain that way. You have to program your brain for health, dynamic, regeneration in order to reverse disease. Healing begins here and this creates that universal energy where you can literally rebuild cells faster than you're destroying them but how do you do that? Movement, intonation, body language, breathing, and I've got to tell you it's the only way to do it.

If you're a calm quiet person, great. But you've got to change your intonation. You've got to change it. This is an exercise. We have to break you out of your shell there. The only way to do it is to start breathing, setting goals, looking at your vision board, and your mind controls cell production. You change your mindset, you change your self-talk, you change the outcome, you actually can reverse disease. Follow the exercises we're giving you and enjoy life.

NOTES

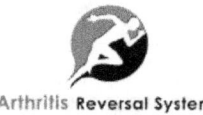

NOTES

NOTES

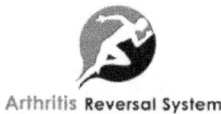

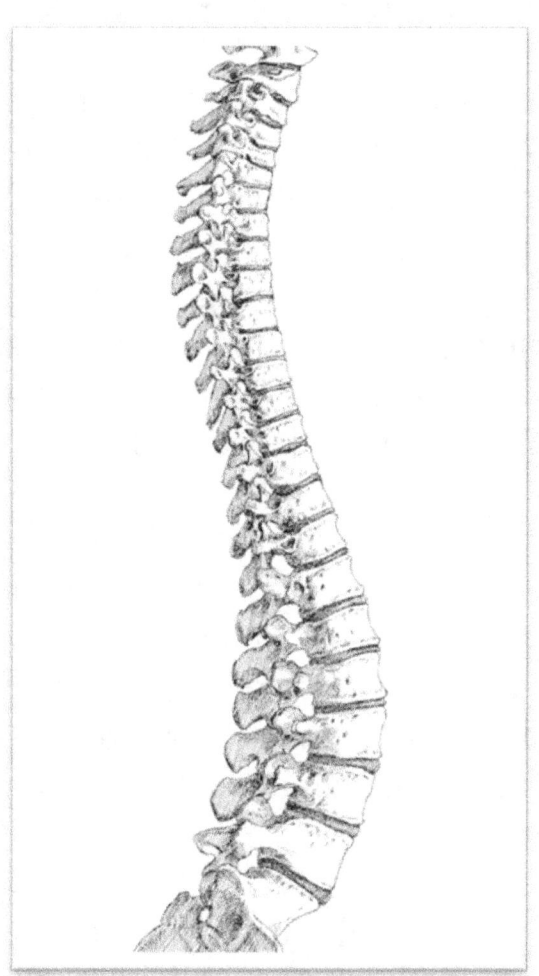

THE NERVOUS SYSTEM

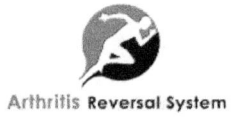

THE NERVOUS SYSTEM

The nervous system. Now this is probably the most exciting organ system that you could possibly have. See, you live your life through your nervous system. What I mean by that is you experience life through your five senses. The way that that information gets to the brain is through the nervous system. You've got pinpoint accuracy on this. I mean, can you touch yourself any spot and not feel it? Not if you have a healthy nervous system. That's the brilliance of this.

The nervous system is actually encased in bone. What a brilliant design. You've got the brain up here that's a solid bone case (skull). And then you've got the spinal cord down here. Now the spinal cord is very delicate so it's protected by this beautiful mobile covering called the spinal column. Now you've got these nerves that are coming off the side that are called peripheral nerves. Now the peripheral nerves are vital.

We're going to talk and mainly focus in on the automatic nervous system. See, the automatic nervous system or the autonomic nervous system is an actual organ system in here. You can see it. In fact, it goes from the top of the rib cage to the bottom of the rib cage, just about. And that's called the fight or flight or sympathetic nervous system. Now the parasympathetic nervous system is called cranial-sacral. So that's the top and the base of the spine. So these are actual organ systems.

PARASYMPATHETIC

Now, it's important that you understand that there's a balance in between the nervous systems. See, your body generates a billion

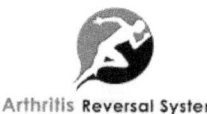

cells a day. That's a billion cells a day. You make most of those when you're under the parasympathetic nervous system or the rest, digest, and repair mode. So to regenerate your body, to reverse disease, to have that healthy dynamic function, you need the parasympathetic nervous system.

SYMPATHETIC

Okay, now you also need the sympathetic nervous system, or the fight or flight to keep you alive short term. This is what gives you the energy; this is how you get your drive. But if you have an imbalance in those systems, that's when disease results [Dis-ease].

Now, under any physical, chemical, emotional stress your body doesn't know the difference, it responds the exact same way to all three. So does that mean if you're emotionally upset, that's the same thing as getting into a traffic accident? It is, as far as your nervous system is concerned. You're going to have the same physiological responses to that.

So that means that under fight or flight...now think of this, if you're being chased by a tiger, you have a stressful circumstance. Do you want blood going to digestion or do you want blood going to arms and legs? Yeah, arms and legs. So does that mean under sympathetic dominance [fight or flight system] does that mean under stress the blood supply to the gut is shut down? Yes, it does. Also, now do you want a lot of light coming into your eyes if you're scared or a little light? A lot. You need to be aware of your surroundings to detect any threats.

See, when I was teaching anatomy I'd say to these young doctors, "What's the connection between the hand and the eye?" So, they got kind of scared. So I'd pick somebody with light colored eyes and I would pinch them on the hand and I'd go, "One, two, three,"

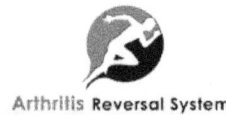

and I'd pinch and I'd cause discomfort. And you could literally see his eyes dilate. The pupils in his eyes dilate. And I've got to tell you, these young doctors would go, "Wow."

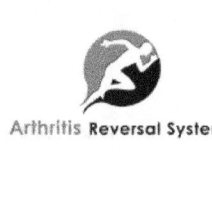

NOTES

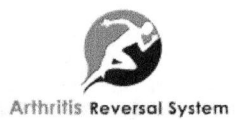

What's the Connection?

So what's the connection, not just between the hand and the eye, what I did was I stimulated, I caused a discomfort, a pain. I put him under stress. So I said, "What did we just do to that guy?" Well, we dilated his pupils. Did we shut blood supply down to the gut? Absolutely we did. So if he had that chronic irritation, that chronic sympathetic dominance, that chronic fight or flight, will he have digestive disorders? Absolutely. If you're trying to repair poor digestion, you're never going to do it if you're sympathetic dominant. It's impossible .

Also, if you're under stress, do you want a lot of energy or a little energy? I've got to tell you, a lot of energy. So your liver's going to break glycogen down to glucose as well. Now, might you get injured if you're in a stress circumstance? Yeah, absolutely. So what happens is your cholesterol goes up. Because cholesterol is the precursor to stress hormones. It's also used for tissue repair. Also, your adrenals produce the greatest anti-inflammatory called cortisol under stress. So this means cortisol is secreted, thyroid function is down, the liver starts to produce more glycogen and glucose so blood sugar goes up, blood pressure, do you think it goes up or down? Well think about this. You're in a stress state. You're in a stress state, do you want a lot of blood pressure or a little blood pressure? You want a lot.

Does that mean, think of this, let's look at this like detectives. So does that mean if you have a chronic sympathetic dominant system, digestive disorders, elevations in blood sugar, elevations in blood pressure, elevations in blood cholesterol. Wow. It kind of opens up that whole idea that if there's physical, chemical, or emotional stress, the autonomic nervous system has an intelligent

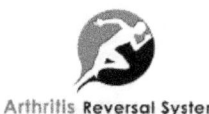

response to that stress, is going to develop those stress responses. So does that mean high blood pressure, type 2 diabetes, cholesterol, digestive disorders that that's not pathology? That it's actually the body adapting to stress? It really does. It really does.

BACK TO THE REST & DIGEST

Now, let's look at the parasympathetic nervous system. The parasympathetic is called the rest, digest and repair mode. And this is why when we talk about visualization and changing your thought patterns and changing, filling your brain, that's when the parasympathetic nervous system kicks in. This is why if you're taking sleep medications that interrupts the rapid eye movement or the deep sleep at night. So, at nighttime, that's when the parasympathetic nervous system kicks in. So you build a billion cells a day. If you're healthy. That means that you're going to destroy a billion cells a day, too.

So you've got this balance of cell destruction and cell repair. Cell destruction and cell repair. If you break down faster than you build up, you have a *dis-ease*. I know, do you like that little hyphen? You have a dis-ease. So the trick is being able to build your body as fast as it breaks down. Then you have health. And what controls that is the parasympathetic nervous system. And you've got to figure that this nervous system, there's so many clues to an imbalance, that if the nervous system isn't right.

And I know it sounds crazy, but today in modern society you're talking that a lot of medical therapies, medical professionals are treating a sympathetic response, a fight or flight response as if it's pathology. That's not pathology, that's the body adapting to physical, chemical or emotional stress. So the stress responses, okay, that most healthcare professionals are treating now are from

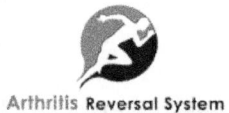

physical, chemical or emotional stress and that causes the sympathetics to be high. So we have to start rethinking this.

NOTES

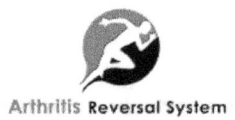

New Way of Thinking

See, if you're prescribed a medication for high blood pressure, high blood sugar, high cholesterol. You've got to rethink this, that perhaps it's a normal response to a sympathetic dominant, or a stressed state.

Now, let's look at the parasympathetic. This is the most brilliant, brilliant part of the nervous system. This regenerates your tissues. Now that's located again at the cranial sacral area. So can you imagine if someone is working at a desk all day long do you think that's going to remodel their spine? Absolutely, pressure over time. This is why movement is so essential to changing how your body functions or how your brain functions.

We can also look at this, you need a balance of those nervous systems for even sexual function. We call it point and shoot. So parasympathetic is the initial phase of an arousal. The shoot is the climactic phase of arousal. So if you have a dysfunction in that area, again *it's the nervous stem*.

Now the nervous system controls digestion, so does this mean most digestive complaints have a nervous system component? Absolutely. Heck, when we know that brain transmitters, one of the most popular ones is serotonin, 90 percent of it is produced in the gut. So does this mean you've got to have healthy digestions for a healthy nervous system function? Wow, you do! People are even calling the gut area the **gut brain**, because it's so intimately involved in how your brain functions, but also impulse control, that's in the frontal lobe.

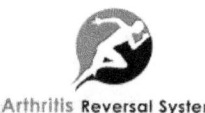

And this is super important because you figure we're talking about the nervous system and I know I'm bringing up diet, I know I'm bringing up adrenals, I know I'm bringing up thyroid, but it's all connected. Okay, now this is super important . How many people have impulse control issues? Well, when we look at the brain itself, there's a lobe called the frontal lobe and this is involved in impulse control, and this is how poor diets can negatively affect the nervous system. If you've been given vaccinations or antibiotics or processed, refined foods, these are actually foods that can blow holes in the intestinal tract. If you have holes in the intestinal tract, large undigested proteins can get into the bloodstream, particularly glutens and caseins, and this comes from toxic grains and say, toxic dairy products.

Well, undigested proteins in the bloodstream actually cause the body to develop an allergic response to it. Or you build antibodies towards it. Now these glutens and caseins can actually attach to the central nervous system, or the frontal lobe. They can literally starve the body. They attach to opiate centers throughout the brain. So, you'll see kids with attention deficit disorder or attention deficit hyperactivity disorder and even autistic kids, kids with mental injures, you're going to see that they crave Mac and Cheese, they crave gluten and dairy because it attaches to the pleasure centers of the brain. However, with it attached up there, it starves the brain.

NOTES

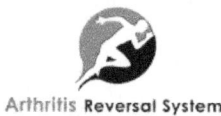

Alternative Source of Brain Power

Now the brain, since the brain controls and coordinates every function of the body, the brain burns glucose, now that's a healthy brain. Well the brain can switch over to a fat metabolism. This is why we recommend medium chain fats or coconut oils or palm oils to help heal the brain damage in dementia, Alzheimer's, autism, attention deficit disorder, all the mental disorders. You have to feed the brain; you have to get the brain healthy.

Now you also have to have that balance. Now, if you have chronic stress, this is where your meditation comes in, this is where your visualization comes in. This is where movement comes in. Because movement, again, the brain is charged like a battery, through normal position and motion of the vertebrae. So if you're stuck in one position, say an office cubicle, oh, there's a nightmare, and you're working all day long, the brain is not getting appropriate stimulus, so this is going to put you in a chronic fight or flight state. So movement is essential.

This is why we see every program that involves movement or exercise is better than any antidepressant drug out there. So look at movement to change and alter brain function. Look at diet to change and alter brain function. Look at stimulus, any type of mental stimulus or mental injury that you can do that will also change that environmental stimulus.

NOTES

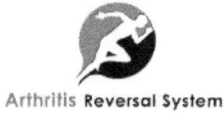

Chronic Stress

Now, under chronic stress, now we've got to go back to the thyroid when we're talking about the nervous system. You've got the thyroid then you've got the adrenals. Thyroid and adrenals. How many people are misdiagnosed with a low functioning thyroid? Because when the adrenals are up, the thyroid's going to appear low. When they thyroid's up, the adrenals are going to appear low. So there has to be a balance. So when we look at this what causes that balance? It's the nervous system. The nervous system controls the pituitary, that controls the thyroid. The nervous system controls the adrenal glands, that controls the hormones.

So, to have a healthy nervous system, to actually make sure it's functioning correctly, you've got to check the joints. And this is why you've got to see a corrective chiropractor in order to make sure that you have appropriate curves, that your body is in alignment because that absolutely affects nervous system, it's called afferentation or sensory input to the brain. You change the input to the brain, you change the control of the brain to the body. You change the input to the brain, you change the control of the brain to the body.

The more you understand that you feed the brain through what you see, what you feel, what you move, okay, and what you envision. See, your thoughts can actually change brain function. And it's interesting, too, that we've seen cortisol levels, and we're talking very high cortisol levels which means a person is under extreme stress. You can reduce cortisol levels by half in most people within about *15 minutes* with deep breathing and meditation. So, your body responds very quickly to appropriate influences. Very quickly.

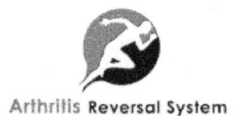

So what I want you to do is start getting your nervous system checked, and this is primary when you're dealing with any disease. The doctor of the future, when he looks at you and finds high blood pressure, high blood sugar, high blood cholesterol, altered mental function, poor digestion, first thing you're going to do with virtually every disease out there is get the nervous system checked and by checked, the only way to check it is to get x-rays to make sure it's in alignment, then you have to check it's influence on the body.

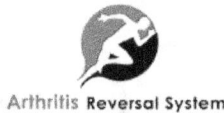

7 Questions

You should have the 7 Questions to Find a Corrective Chiropractor in your packet. Here is a quick reminder:

1. Do you take x-rays?

2. Do you get spinal listings off of the x-rays? (some Doctors only take x-rays because they can bill for them)

3. Is your goal to restore normal function or only symptom relief? (Most Doctors: MD's, DC's, Physical therapists treat only symptoms and that is NOT Corrective care)

4. Do you take post x-rays to document the structural changes made? (This is the only way to show correction)

5. Are you familiar with repairing disc injuries? (this requires a high level of skill)

6. Do you work with post spinal surgery patients? (this requires a high level of skill)

7. Do you work with Pediatrics and the Elderly? (this requires very specific techniques)

NOTES

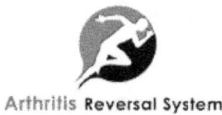

Additional Studies

We use a heart rate variability study. And you could also check it with a rolling thermal scan; you could also check it with surface electromyography to see how the brain is adapting to your body's position in space. But you need one of those four tests or all four of them to make sure that the nervous system is working correctly and you're getting correct influences to the brain because I've got to tell you, if your nervous system is off [I shift my body to the side], like mine is now, this is altering my function to the brain, this is altering sensory input to the brain, it's going to alter the way my brain controls my body, it's going to put me in either a sympathetic or parasympathetic dominant state. It's going to keep me in chronic fight or flight mode or chronic rest and digest mode where I won't have any energy, I won't have any motivation.

In the afternoon, if someone's stuck in a parasympathetic dominant state, at the end of the day, they are done. Man, 3:00, 4:00 in the afternoon rolls around and they want to take a nap. And there's no incentive, there's no vibrancy, there's no spark. If someone's in the parasympathetic dominant stage, they start to break down, their tissue breaks down, they don't have the resistance to disease, their body ages before their time. So we've got to have balance.

When you're talking about the nervous system, balance of the parasympathetic and sympathetic, you don't want to eliminate stress. You want to be able to handle the physical, chemical and emotional stressors in a healthy fashion. The only people that don't have stress, they're in the graveyard. Stress keeps you alive, stress keeps you strong, stress keeps you healthy and focused. However, if you can't handle stress correctly, it can kill you. So,

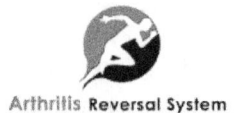

you live your life through your nervous system. Get your nervous system checked, primarily by a corrective chiropractor.

NOTES

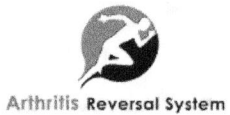

MDs Don't Look for what they Can't Fix

And what's tough is, see a lot of medical professions out there, a lot of health care professionals, if they can't fix it; they're not going to look for it. It's kind of like me working on a transmission. I know at D, the car goes forward, the R, it goes backwards.

It's the same way when a medical doctor looks at a spine on an x-ray. If they see a reverse curve in the neck, they have no tools to fix it. They might send you over to an orthopedic surgeon; however, we're talking over *80 percent failure rate* on surgeries. So if they see a reverse curve in the neck, the doctor of the future will actually say, "Wow you've got a reverse curve of the neck, we need to get you to a corrective chiropractor quickly and restore that and then that's going to alter your physiology down to a normal state and your body's going to be able to adapt and you can now reverse the disease that you're experiencing." That's the doctor of the future.

The doctor of the future will look at the nervous system, realizing that high blood pressure, high cholesterol, digestive disorders and you're talking altered mental function, all of those, high cholesterol, all of those disease states are not disease states. They're the body adapting to physical, chemical and emotional stress.

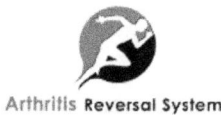

SUMMARY & CALL TO ACTION

So we balance out that nervous system, you check that nervous system primary. When we talk about reversing arthritis, you've got to check the nervous system first. Why? That controls digestion. It controls the nutrients in your system. It controls how the body can regenerate itself. How you break those proteins to amino acids, the fats to the fatty essence, the carbohydrates to the usable sugars. Your nervous system controls that, nothing else.

Get your nervous system checked. And please, study how your body works and appreciate it. Your body is more energy than matter and that energy flows from the brain down. Healing occurs from above, down, inside out. And that's been true since slime formed on a pond. Healing occurs from the inside out.

In a human being, the most brilliant biologic structure the world's ever seen, healing occurs from the brain down, from the inside out. We have this downstream, outside in philosophy where we're going to introduce drugs to change the nervous system, we're going to introduce pills or potions or lotions. That is crazy. Because your body is rarely ever suffering a deficiency of Tylenol or a deficiency of Advil or a deficiency of a beta blocker or diuretic. That doesn't make sense. Respect the body first. And this goes to all the health care professionals out there as well.

Look at why the symptom is there, because you live your life through your nervous system and that nervous system is doing it's best job to tell you if it's sympathetic or parasympathetic dominant, if there's some type of alterations in brain function, you change the brain, you change the nervous system, you change the outcome of

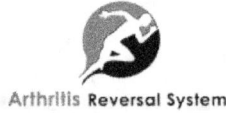

your life, you actually achieve optimum health and disease reversal.

Make sure you write down in your journals, what you're eating, what you're meditating on, how your exercise program is going. Make sure that you take accurate notes, replay these tapes back so that you can own it. The more you understand how your body works, and we're going to be helping you along this, you are going to be amazed at how fast you regenerate.

NOTES

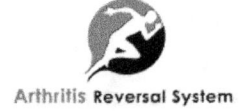

NOTES

NOTES

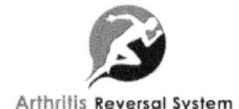

www.ingramcontent.com/pod-product-compliance
Lightning Source LLC
Chambersburg PA
CBHW080252180526
45167CB00006B/2507